Travels with Shubh

iUniverse, Inc.
New York   Bloomington

Travels with Shubh

A Memoir of the MetaWorks Journey

iUniverse books may be ordered through booksellers or by contacting:

iUniverse
1663 Liberty Drive
Bloomington, IN 47403
www.iuniverse.com
1-800-Authors (1-800-288-4677)

ISBN: 978-1-4401-5261-0 (pbk)
ISBN: 978-1-4401-5262-7 (ebk)

Printed in the United States of America

iUniverse rev. date: 9/17/2009

Travels with Shubh:

A Memoir of the MetaWorks Journey

Susan Ross, MD

Contents

Acknowledgments

I wish to thank all those mentioned in this memoir, and many more unmentioned, for their help and inspiration in making the MetaWorks dream come true. In particular, I thank Dr. Thomas Chalmers for his sparkling brilliance and his most generous mentoring. I thank all my talented and feisty colleagues at MetaWorks who skillfully crewed our little ship, day in and day out. I thank my husband for his never-failing optimism, without which this journey may never have begun. And lastly, I thank my power-trio partners: Janet, for her strength and constancy, from beginning to end; and, of course, Shubh, the happy lens through which this MetaWorks history is viewed. And while I am grateful and indebted for their support of MetaWorks and, directly or indirectly, their support of this book, I am solely responsible for any errors or lapses that appear herein.

1. Introduction

In this country, it takes ten to fifteen years to bring a new drug to market. For every five thousand compounds that enter preclinical testing, only one ever makes it all the way through the gauntlet to win full approval by the Food and Drug Administration (FDA). This ridiculous attrition rate, plus the need to develop bulletproof evidence in support of each new drug application, contributes to the stratospheric costs of bringing a new drug to market: $800 million, on average, at last estimate.

It was MetaWorks' founding contention that these figures—indicative of both time and money—represent grossly unnecessary waste. Yet the pharmaceutical industry back in the early 1990s had little motivation to change its ways, as long as profits were also at record highs. Only when those profits have been threatened, as they are now, have we seen profound industry changes under way. Formerly "fat, dumb, and happy" drug companies have been scrutinized, criticized, pushed, prodded, pulled, and in some cases, dragged kicking and screaming into the smarter, faster, and less forgiving information age. The good-times culture of throwaway assets, particularly information assets, is no longer tenable for long-term survival, let alone prosperity.

In 1993, MetaWorks was founded to "harness the power of data." We understood then that information in drug development and commercialization was a fundamental, yet neglected, corporate asset. We believed that this information flows like a mighty river fed by countless tributaries—mostly uncharted and untapped. We were explorers on this river. What follows is the story of the MetaWorks voyage and of the many wonderful, and some not so wonderful, people we met along the way. The story unfolds through the mantras of one unique MetaWorker in particular, named Shubh, who, in bad times, somehow made it bearable, and in good times, made it all so much fun.

2. The Idea

In the summer of 1992, I went to rural Ontario for a week's vacation. I brought along a few dozen medical journals that I was going to read. Like everyone else in medicine, I never had enough time to keep current with my journal reading. I counted on using vacations for catch-up time. But I knew in my heart that even if I had all the time in the world, I'd still never be able to keep up. I'd be drowning in information. It's been estimated that if a specialist were to read one new study per day every single day, then after one year, she'd be about twelve years behind the current literature in her field!

Ignoring the obvious futility of my task, very early each morning, before the rest of the household roused, I would sit out on the sunny, open deck at the back of our farmhouse with lots of coffee and the occasional hummingbird as my only company. I would flip through journal after journal, trolling for items of interest. I still remember the jolt that hit me as I scanned one article in particular, in the *New England Journal of Medicine*, about a meta-analysis of studies of streptokinase (a clot busting drug) in patients with heart attacks. I recall that hallelujah moment as I realized how remarkable this article really was. It wasn't the streptokinase story per se that grabbed me, but rather the challenge its authors posed to all readers—clinicians, investigators, drug companies—to get smarter about the way we use information in medicine. The paper fairly shouted: "Wake up! We are all sitting on mountains of data that could answer so many of our questions in medicine. So why aren't we *using* it?"

3

I ripped the article out of the journal, thinking, "This one's a keeper." Then, as if to drive the point home, I next picked up a recent edition of the *Journal of the American Medical Association* (*JAMA*), which contained, lo and behold, a companion article by the same authors! The gist of this one was that the statistical tool called meta-analysis could be applied to mountains of clinical data to make better sense of it. Examples were given of how meta-analysis of existing data could have pointed the way to many safe and effective treatments years before the usual experts finally got around to recommending them.

It was clear these guys were on to something desperately needed in medicine. Their message could be applicable to anyone making decisions in health care about insurance coverage, health policy, patient care, and pharmaceutical research and development. I resolved to get in touch with the senior author on both papers, Dr. Thomas Chalmers of the Harvard School of Public Health, as soon as I returned from vacation. And I did. And that is how MetaWorks got started.

In those days, Hillary Clinton was busy "reforming" health care, and Al Gore had recently "invented" the Internet. People were beginning to talk about the information explosion in the biological and clinical sciences. Journals were starting to publish online, with all the unlimited space for data that medium affords. Progress in sequencing the human genome was on an accelerating curve, and biotech was a brave new industry. With the convergence of these trends and needs, it seemed the perfect time to introduce new ways of doing things in medicine, to introduce a technique and a mindset that challenged outmoded assumptions and inefficiencies in using data to answer questions, and to reduce uncertainty in decision making.

MetaWorks would be the child of an unprecedented marriage of statistics and medicine. This may not seem like a revolutionary idea now, but back then, it was still a very unique proposition. To introduce more quantitative analytic methods to the art of medicine was considered heretical by many. Evidence-based medicine was new wave, and most clinicians initially resisted it as either the trendy ravings of a few British and Canadian (i.e., Socialist) fanatics, or, even worse, as "cookbook" medicine pushed by American businessmen to protect the bottom line. The practice of medicine has always been a varying blend of facts and intuition. Could or should an explicit, analytical approach to diagnosis and treatment decisions replace the ancient and elegant art of medicine? It's disconcerting, nay, threatening, to have established practices challenged on the basis of evidence or lack thereof.

A perfect case in point was the now-famous lidocaine example from Chalmers' *JAMA* paper. Lidocaine was used reflexively in the coronary care unit when I was a medical resident. If a patient with a heart attack developed life-threatening ventricular arrhythmias, he got lidocaine. It worked, too. But what had not been demonstrated until Chalmers came along was that survival of patients receiving lidocaine was actually lower than of patients with the same problems but not receiving lidocaine. In other words, with lidocaine, you might succeed in suppressing the arrhythmia, but the patient might die anyway. You could win the battle but lose the war. In fact, Chalmers showed that such patients might be *more* likely to die with lidocaine. This was a disruptive notion for most physicians who had practiced in coronary care units. It was counter-intuitive. Yet it was true. We didn't know this before, because we hadn't thought to ask the question. Even if we had asked, we didn't know enough to apply the statistical tool of meta-analysis to the large amount of data that was out there; as long as these data were scattered and unexamined, they were useless. The true answer became apparent only when consider-ing *all* the relevant information together, as a whole that is greater than the sum of its parts. This was the seductive power and beauty of meta-analysis—elegant, iconoclastic, possibly dangerous, and simply irresistible.

But let's back up for a moment. Meta-analysis as a statistical tool had been around for decades, with accepted applications in the fields of agriculture, envi-ronmental science, and the social sciences. But not until the 1980s was its promise in medicine first appre-ciated. In 1985, Ingram Olkin of Stanford University, along with Richard Hedges at the University of Chicago, wrote the preeminent reference book on the principles and methods of meta-analysis. Around the same time, Richard Peto and colleagues in the UK showed how important this technique could be in answering ques-tions about the management of patients with breast cancer. Thomas Chalmers ran with the idea, stateside, to fulfill the promise of meta-analysis in medicine. The remarkable twin set of articles in the *New England Journal of Medicine* and *JAMA* have since been lauded as seminal publications of twentieth-century medicine. Why? Because they challenged the medical profession to think differently.

3. Thinking Differently

When I first met Dr. Thomas Chalmers, he told me about his six careers in medicine. He was first a clinician, a practicing gastroenterologist. He was also a clinical researcher. Then, he was in medical administration at the VA hospital in Roxbury, Massachusetts. He had also served in the federal government in the upper echelons of the National Institutes of Health (NIH). He then had accepted the presidency of Mt. Sinai Hospital in New York City. And after that, he returned to Boston to head the Technology Assessment Group at the Harvard School of Public Health. It's a good thing I didn't know all this in the summer of '92, or I might never have had the nerve to pick up the phone to call him, to invite him to embark on what would be his seventh career.

But, as it was, I was blissfully ignorant about him, and I could hardly wait for my summer vacation to be over, so I could call him. As soon as I returned to Boston, I tracked down his phone number at the Harvard School of Public Health. I did worry about what to say to him and how to say it. Would he, a big-shot Harvard professor, deign to speak to me? Might I lack the necessary credentials to be taken seriously? After all, I wasn't from Harvard. I had no academic affiliations to speak of. I had no claim to fame. And worse, I had worked in "industry." Would he consider me thereby tainted, and would he judge me in the same deprecating way I used to judge drug company doctors who hosted free lunches at my old teaching hospital?

I decided I had nothing to lose but my dignity, so I

forced myself to dial his number. To my amazement, he was not only civil during our first phone conversation, but actually friendly ("call me Tom") and interested. So I suggested we meet to discuss some ideas I had for real-world applications of his work. He gave me an appointment. Then, I hastily worked with my husband and his brother—both local businessmen—to try to prepare an outline of a business model I could understand well enough to present persuasively to the great man. I needed a believable rationale to convince him to leave academia and work in the private sector.

On the appointed day, we found him in the basement of the School of Public Health building, crammed into a gloomy and claustrophobic warren of windowless offices. I was surprised to see that Harvard shut up its stars in dungeons like this, for not only was Tom holed up down there, but so were Dr. Graham Colditz and Dr. Frederick Mosteller. In the fields of medicine, statistics, and public health, these guys were among the brightest stars in the firmament of notables—and here they worked, shut up in the hot and airless bowels of a building on Huntington Avenue. As Tom showed us to his office, he apologized for the surroundings and said he wasn't going to be there for long, as he had already decided to "defect," to take a better opportunity where he'd be better appreciated, at a rival institution across town.

He was tall and lean, with kind eyes, a quick and easy smile, and a neat white mustache. He wore the Ivy League uniform of tweed jacket and bow tie with casual confidence. He offered me an overhead projector for my transparencies—this was before the days of PowerPoint—and seated his hastily assembled colleagues to hear me out. They listened politely, and I answered a few questions. Tom then stood up and, without further discussion, pronounced judgment: this was a good idea, and we should do it. And that's how he was ever after—easy to be around, optimistic, confident, and always willing to think differently.

He was also always scrupulously forthcoming. As he escorted us back outside, he confided, "If we're going to work together on this, there's something you should know about me. I have prostate cancer. It's in remission, and I feel great, but you never know how long this will last. I don't know how long I'll be able to do this with you."

We assured him we were willing to chance it, as long as he was. He smiled, we all shook hands, and the good ship MetaWorks was effectively launched.

4.   Getting Real on State Street

Tom's new office at Tufts/New England Medical Center was a lot nicer than his Harvard office. This one, although also crowded, was upstairs, with windows that let in fresh air and sunshine.   One huge advantage for Tom was the helpful physical proximity of his meta-analyst collaborator at Tufts, Dr. Joseph Lau. When we original MetaWorkers needed to meet, we'd all squeeze into Tom's new office. We'd plan our strategy, discuss our future customers and our future services, and make lists of our future staff, using names from our respective Rolodexes to recruit.   It was a light and hopeful time, still unburdened by the weight of running a real company. But it was clear that if we were ever going to be a real company, we'd have to get a real office somewhere soon.

This was to be our first concrete commitment in more ways than one. We now had to assume a real financial risk, our first of many. We signed a lease for an office suite in an old building on State Street, next to the Custom House tower. We loved all the unaccustomed space. We loved having our own address. We admired our beautiful new logo, which was the color of the sea in March, and our spiffy new letterhead. It still felt like play.

The only damper to our new office fun was the fact that we had to share our third floor with a steady stream of visitors to a mysterious clinic at the end of the hall. We noticed an unusual number of hollow-eyed street people riding up and down the elevator with us. And it was not unusual to find some pretty wasted-looking people in our shared washrooms, peeing into little bottles and leaving them on the edge of the sink, from which they would later mysteriously disappear. We wondered if somehow we'd rented office space in the middle of a methadone clinic or worse. And we worried about the impression this could have on our future customers, were they to visit us. Evidently, we were doing business in the low-rent section of Boston's financial district, but one to which the local color lent significant hip cachet. However, it didn't last long. In less than two years, we'd outgrown the rough office space we'd grown to love. Although we had had to squeeze in two, and sometimes three MetaWorkers, to a room, the rabbit warren effect was cozy and conducive to frequent laughter. We were still riding high, with no wrong turns and no casualties yet to deal with.

Our early growth spurt was due to the early adoption of our services by a market sector that took us by surprise: the pharmaceutical industry. In our original thinking about which health care stakeholders would need the types of research syntheses we offered, we listed insurers and managed care groups, the government, formularies, health care policy makers, Wall Street investors, everyday clinicians and institutional health care providers, academic researchers, and even consumers. Drug companies were way down at the bottom of the list. In fact, we designed our MetaWorks logo to signify a hub of data from which numerous information products and services would spin out, to serve all those health care constituencies.

Moreover, we fully intended to do well by doing good. In that spirit, we preferred to offer our services to those who were closer to patient care. Both Tom and I wanted nothing less than to change the practice of medicine from one based too often on intuition, outdated opinion, and anecdote, to one based upon data that was explicitly collected and analyzed and critically appraised. As it turns out, these are pretty much the same motives that drove the "Evidence-based Medicine" movement, which was just getting under way around the same time we were starting MetaWorks. To get the word out to clinicians, insurers, managed care directors, and formulary managers, we attended professional and trade meetings, sent out letters, and followed up with phone calls. The best response we got was polite interest, always qualified by a plea of insufficient funds. This was hard to believe, since at the time, the managed care industry, for one, was reaping enormous profits—mostly by managing expenses, not by managing care, as it turned out. We soon learned that everyone paid lip service to the value of having better information to make decisions, but no one wanted to pay for it. No one, that is, except drug companies. They had deep pockets, and they alone were willing to put their money on the line. And MetaWorks *was* supposed to be a business. So, like Willie Sutton, we, too, followed the money.

There's a saying in clinical trials that the first patient enrolled always does really well, but subsequent patients never do as well again. First swing at bat, you hit a home run, but after that, you struggle mightily for each and every single. So it was with our first few "patients", a.k.a. pharma customers. We won their business almost too easily. But, of course, we didn't know that then. Only with the help of the retrospectoscope can I see how easy it was for us to get the comfortable (and slightly deluded) sense that there was a huge untapped business opportunity out there just waiting for us to grab: the proverbial low-hanging fruit. We really believed that "if we build it, they will come." Still, we were lucky to have that early success, for without the encouragement of those first few pharmaceutical industry customers, we might not have found the resources to persist as long as we did.

Schering Plough was among those early adopters, identified as a result of a cheap little tabletop exhibit we set up at a small meeting of health services researchers in Washington. We handed out a crude little pamphlet about MetaWorks. And I mean crude. I know, because I pasted a picture from a Microsoft Clip Art menu, wrote a brief text blurb, printed it on a black and white printer on 8½ × 11 inch white paper, and folded it in half for mailings and distribution at meetings. Such was our first official MetaWorks brochure.

Nevertheless, it was some combination of that excellent material and my businessman brother-in-law's powers of persuasion that brought us one of our first real projects from Schering Plough. We performed a systematic review of the literature on all clinical uses of interferon alpha. At the time, this product was officially approved by the FDA for use in about six clinical conditions, but we soon discovered by plowing through the literature that it was being tested by investigators around the world for over sixty different diseases. With the "geological survey" map we produced from this vast literature, we were able to recommend to the customer where they might consider "drilling for oil" (i.e., where there appeared to be a sufficient amount and quality of published evidence of the efficacy and safety of interferon alpha) We were most gratified subsequently when this same client did, in fact, "drill for oil." They pursued supplemental label indications at the FDA for interferon alpha in two cancers suggested by our survey, and supported by the meta-analyses we were subsequently able to produce using articles already in the published literature.

Drug companies still request these "geological surveys" of the existing evidence in the public domain. For certain marketed products, the value of a map of the evidence for marketing and regulatory purposes is obvious. And the "sell" is simple: why spend zillions of dollars to do a new trial to support a new clinical indication, when, in fact, there already exists plenty of adequate and well-controlled evidence of efficacy and safety?

Another early adopting pharma company was AstraMerck, as it was then called, who asked us to use existing evidence to build a case for the use of omeprazole, the first marketed proton pump inhibitor, in treating people with peptic ulcers. Given the fact that no one argues this point anymore—and you can even buy proton pump inhibitors over the counter—you may think this was a silly undertaking. But that was a different time. A brave (or crazy) Australian scientist had recently, intentionally, imbibed a cocktail laced with a nasty little microorganism called *Helicobacter pylori* to prove his hypothesis that peptic ulcers were caused by *Helicobacter* infection. The age-old approach to treating peptic ulcers had been turned upside down, and there was a lot of new uncertainty about which medications to use to achieve ulcer healing and *Helicobacter* eradication. So the role of omeprazole was still quite unknown.

The multidisciplinary AstraMerck team believed that omeprazole had an important role to play and that a credible third party group like MetaWorks, particularly with a gastroenterologist and world-class meta-analyst rolled into one, might be the best group to pull together the existing evidence, meta-analyze it if possible, and publish it. We were only too pleased to help them out. This was one of those early projects that fell into our laps simply because of Tom's reputation. And it clearly helped us to build our corporate foundations, both financial and procedural. But what a painful project it became. The customer's team members and their project objectives changed repeatedly over the subsequent months. We had to change project direction, including numerous redos of work, several times. And on top of that, the published data were a mess; they were "dirty," inconsistent, and full of holes. These burdens, we've subsequently learned, are common to most research syntheses of the literature.

Our third early client was Pfizer. In 1995, Pfizer was in trouble. A crisis had been precipitated by two separate but nearly concurrent publications that had questioned the safety of one of Pfizer's top selling drugs, a calcium channel blocker called nifedipine. Although nifedipine alone had been incriminated, a pall had been cast over all calcium channel blockers. And Pfizer had another, newer calcium channel blocker, amlodipine, in its stable, which promised to be a bigger blockbuster than nifedipine. One of these incriminating publications was an epidemiologic study, and one was a meta-analysis. When Pfizer brass decided to fight data with data, they decided to find the nation's top meta-analyst in medicine. They found Tom Chalmers. Their author search of the literature turned up hundreds of publications with Tom's name on them, including numerous meta-analyses. So they came to the source and asked us to perform a meta-analysis of the literature. We told them we were happy to do this as long as we had full control of the entire process. No problem, they told us.

There *was* one big problem, however. We were asked to produce this meta-analysis in only six weeks. It was needed for an FDA document with an immovable submission date. I was too inexperienced in these things to know if this would really be possible, but when they told us their deadline, Tom turned to me and asked, "Can we *do* it that fast?" "Why not?" said I, with unjustified confidence. When you have just started an exciting new company, and you see a high-profile, high-paying opportunity just sitting there for the taking, you grab hold of it, and you make it work. Failure was not an option. Tom turned back to the Pfizer team and announced, "This will be the fastest meta-analysis anyone has ever done!"

Tom called upon a long list of former students and otherwise experienced acquaintances to lend a hand, and soon we had a small army of clinicians and methodologists busy with the many tasks inherent in a systematic review of the literature: writing a project protocol, designing data extraction forms, searching Medline and retrieving papers, and whiting out all investigator and drug identifiers in each accepted paper so as not to introduce any bias in the selection of data elements for extraction. Then we had to create an analyzable database by entering and checking all the study data that our doctors had extracted and consensed. Then, the actual statistical analyses followed, using two accepted methods of meta-analysis, called fixed effects and random effects models. Then, the whole exercise had to be written up in excruciating detail as a final report, so it could be replicated, if need be, by the FDA and anyone else who might read it and care to try. This army of experts marched along behind the project commander, Tom, and we actually met our six-week deadline.

5. Enter Shubh

After the success of the Pfizer project, it seemed that MetaWorks' future, at least in the short term, lay in catering to the enormous information needs of the pharmaceutical industry. They were the first market segment to "get it," and they certainly could afford it. So we concluded that it was high time to develop a professional marketing and sales presence in the pharmaceutical sector. Enter Shubh.

Shubh and I had met years earlier while working together at a local biotech company. We'd both gone our separate ways in the years since then. But when the need for professional marketing arose at MetaWorks, I thought of Shubh immediately. He's not the sort of person you easily forget.

When he was an eighteen-year-old student, Shubh had come to Chicago from his home in northern India. He'd been the youngest of several children of a wealthy family living in the wrong place at the wrong time. When the British left India the late 1940s, at the stroke of a pen, his family's land holdings—nearly all of their assets—had landed on the wrong side of the newly drawn border with Pakistan. His father, then well into his fifties, had been forced to write it all off and start over, managing to amass a second fortune during Shubh's childhood. With his father's example behind him and an older brother beckoning from America, Shubh had come to the land of opportunity. He'd completed his education, holding down several jobs while going to college. He'd married a local girl from rural Illinois, and he'd risen through a series of sales and marketing positions in pharmaceutical companies.

19

What I remembered from our shared biotech experience was an energy, warmth, and sense of humor that could melt the cool reserve of the most uptight New Englander, me included. I just hoped he might still be available and interested in helping out. He was both. Thus began my travels with Shubh.

Our first marketing strategy session was a minor fiasco. Luckily, Shubh was not dissuaded by MetaWorks' business naïveté. The meeting was held in the dining room of my home, which we had equipped with the requisite flip charts and markers. MetaWorks' four founders, namely the two Ross brothers on the business side, and Tom and I on the science side, listened dutifully while Shubh presented his SWOT (he informed us that means "Strengths, Weaknesses, Opportunities, and Threats") analysis of MetaWorks. Then, he enthusiastically led us through his formal plan for our success as an evidence provider to the pharmaceutical industry.

Tom was silent throughout the presentation, pacing all the while around the dining room table. When Shubh concluded, Tom announced, "That's all well and good, but I still don't understand why we *need* a marketing plan!"

Shubh was uncharacteristically speechless. I don't think he'd anticipated any challenges to his core assumptions. But in Tom's world of academic medicine and research, neither business speak nor business practice got much respect. In Boston, in medical academia, "business" itself is suspect, at best, and just plain dirty the rest of the time. But Shubh soldiered on. "MetaWorks *is* a business, Tom. Right? And the purpose of a business is to gain and keep its customers. We can't forget that."

Silence.

Once more, making eye contact with each of us in turn, he repeated very slowly and deliberately, waving his arms like a symphony conductor as he intoned mantra number one: "The purpose of a business is to gain and keep its customers. The purpose of a business is to gain and keep its customers. The purpose of a business is to gain and keep its customers."

6.   Exit Tom

Late in the summer of 1995, Tom invited all MetaWorkers to join other assorted guests at a picnic at his family's compound on Squam Lake in New Hampshire. The movie *On Golden Pond* had been filmed there a few summers earlier, so it held that magical quality of a place you've visited only through the silver screen. I was delighted to stay with my family in "Katherine Hepburn's bungalow." Others stayed in "Henry Fonda's cabin," and the overflow slept in tents, on the porch, and at neighboring motels.

We were treated to a fine Chalmers tradition—randomized wine tasting. The brave and the foolish among us tasted, in randomized sequence, five mystery wines, all with labels removed and bottles wrapped in foil, with quality ranging from ordinary to extraordinary. The scoring for each taster was based on the sum of correct guesses of each wine's pedigree. In many years of running this experiment at Chalmers picnics, the number of tasters who consistently distinguished cheap from expensive wine was laughably low. MetaWorkers were no exception.

The wine tasting was completely in keeping with Tom's iconoclastic approach to answering questions. To discover the fastest way to get to the office, he'd randomly choose different routes to drive, holding other potentially important factors, such as time of day, constant. Then, only the route that was proven to be the fastest would win. Or, to determine whether his dependence upon caffeine was real or just imagined, his wife, Frankie, randomly alternated his morning coffee between decaffeinated and caffeinated brew without telling him which was which. (He correctly identified the caffeinated version.) Or, later, when he needed pain killers for cancer, he wanted to know which pain killer, A or B, worked better for him, so he ran an early "n-of-1" clinical trial with his clinician in New Hampshire. His analgesic was alternated at random, with its identity masked by the prescribing doctor, until Tom could decide whether drug A or B worked better for him. Just as in a clinical trial, the randomization and the masking of choices like these are important ways to reduce bias in assessing different interventions.

Tom did not live to present the findings of our Pfizer meta-analysis to the FDA Cardio-Renal Advisory Committee that convened in January 1996 to review the safety of calcium channel blockers. To everyone's dismay, his cancer had returned with a vengeance late in the fall of 1995. His health deteriorated very rapidly, but he continued to work on double-checking our nifedipine report and preparing our presentation until just days before the end. His MetaWorks assistant, Greg, and I visited him in his New Hampshire hospital room in December, assuming we'd find him in a classic deathbed scene. Instead, he was sitting up in bed, keeping his nurses scurrying back and forth, using his call button mercilessly. He laughed as we surveyed with amazement the stacks of papers on the floor surrounding his bed, on the windowsill, and piled here and there on cabinets and tables all around the edges of the room. He was still planning analyses, still reading studies, and still extracting data.

He died within days of our visit, while still the center

of the busy hive of activity he loved. Once, early on, when his cancer was still in remission, he had told me he hoped he would die quickly, "with his boots on." I'm glad to think he got that wish.

With Tom gone, we had to find a suitable successor, another scientific champion. At Tom's urging, we'd actually begun the search for his successor before his death. He gave us a long list of possible candidates— all academics, all published experts in the field of meta-analysis, and some with more "star quality" than others, but all capable.

We contacted one after another of these people to assess their potential interest in joining MetaWorks as our chief scientist. Most would not even consider it; what we were proposing was just too risky for their professional careers. Nearly all expressed a need to remain in the personal comfort zone of academia. The few exceptions had other issues we could not overcome. In one case, the candidate demanded ownership of a whopping 80 percent of the company in exchange for his joining. Shocked and amused at his chutzpah, we declined. Another candidate (in Canada) decided that he didn't want to raise his family in America. Another had no problem, personally, living in Boston, but his wife would not consider leaving her job in Philadelphia. And so it continued, until, one by one, all twelve candidates were eliminated.

We next decided that, until we could find a scientific champion to replace Tom, MetaWorks would have to get by with a pinch hitter—me. In the three years since I had first met Tom at Harvard, I'd had the opportunity to perform a few systematic reviews with him, working under his direct tutelage. I had coauthored some meeting abstracts, manuscripts, and project proposals with him. I had written standard operating procedures for our reviews and analyses, based upon his methodologies. I had prepared slide presentations with his input. But I did not consider myself an expert in this field. To keep MetaWorks alive, however, I stepped to the plate, bat in hand, full of trepidation.

Lucky for me, and lucky for MetaWorks, Tom had left in place a Scientific Advisory Board, including statistics guru Professor Ingram Olkin from Stanford, and Dr. Bert Spilker, who'd written "the book" (several, actually) on drug development. These advisors, and countless others along the way, proved to be a legacy that kept on giving through all the years that followed.

7. "The Purpose of a Business Is to Gain and Keep Its Customers"

So "if the purpose of a business is to gain and keep its customers," with Shubh as my new business tutor, I immediately found myself on another steep learning curve; this one pertained to the massively complicated pharma sector. I soon learned that drug companies are as varied as trees in a forest. There are slow-growing behemoths and fast-growing young upstarts. They all compete for their share of the sun and water, and every year a few come crashing down in storms or just from internal rot. This natural winnowing is good, because it leaves more room for the remainder to grow.

But maybe the forest is not a perfect analogy, since a forest has thousands of trees, and the pharma industry is really quite finite. I'd guess there are only about thirty companies of any consequence, globally, and only about fifteen to twenty that really matter. But, boy, do they matter. These companies employ thousands of people around the world. They pour billions of dollars every year into the research and development of new drugs—some of which really do make a difference in people's lives, but others of which, unfortunately, are just redundant knock-offs of some other company's innovation, called "me too" drugs in the industry. As such, pharma provides a large portion of all the money that is devoted to research in academia. These companies effectively lobby Congress. If, for some reason you, or Ralph Nader, decide to sue them, you'll probably lose to the crème de la crème of the legal profession in court. They now speak directly to you and me on TV, often through celebrity spokespersons like Dorothy Hamill, Bob Dole, or Cal Ripkin. They "educate" our doctors, both before and long after graduation from medical school. In short, their influence is enormous.

As I mentioned above, the pharma business sector has a finite and shrinking number of big players. They swap partners, occasionally gobble each other up, and occasionally spin off fledgling or flailing companies. As such, the corporate landscape continues to change, but while the companies change, the people remain the same. They just move around, as if in a big, crazy game of musical chairs.

At MetaWorks, we continued to run into the same customers over and over again. Only their company affiliations changed. I'd like to think that these people moved up the corporate ladder because they were so enlightened as to use our services to advance their drug development and commercialization objectives. Use of MetaWorks is a good screening test, so to speak, for successful managers and strategists in the pharma industry.

Of lesser influence, but still a force to be reckoned with, are the smaller and newer trees in the forest: the biotech companies. Not saplings by any means, but still lacking the trunk girth of the Mercks and Pfizers, these companies have been around since the 1980s, and a few of them, like Amgen have grown so fast and so big that they look more like their large pharma cousins than their biotech siblings.

Biotech companies always cultivate the aura of brilliant risk-takers and rebels, and in some cases, I think this is true. Some of the most brilliant advances in biology and medicine this century have been born at the whiteboards or nurtured in the clinical trials of biotech companies, often working in tight collaboration with academics. Examples? Consider anemia, and credit Amgen with recombinant erythropoietin. Consider rheumatoid arthritis, and credit Immunex (now Amgen and Wyeth) for anti-TNF. Consider multiple sclerosis, and credit Biogen for beta-interferon. Consider cancer, and credit IDEC (now Biogen) for anti-CD25 in lymphoma; or credit Genentech for Herceptin in breast cancer.

Unfortunately, success stories like these have also been accompanied by considerable failure. For several years in the 1990s, if you were a so-called "biotech" company with an idea, no matter how ridiculous, you could raise a lot of money if you had a good storyteller on your side. If you could make a decent "pitch," you could raise tons of cash. Then, if you were like lots of other biotech "NewCos," you could spend money indiscriminately for a couple of years and have a whale of a time doing it. A ridiculous amount of venture money has been wasted on fancy executive suites, first class travel and hotels, gourmet meals, and cultivation of influential "friends" in Washington and "advisors" in academia. Only a few biotechs have stood the test of time, however, and not necessarily those with better science or more money. The survivors are the companies with the best management.

And then there is the whole support industry catering to all those pharma and biotech companies. This is where MetaWorks fits into the industry picture. Just take a stroll through the exhibit floor of any annual meeting of the Drug Information Association (DIA)— the industry trade show—and you will find hundreds of little companies that only exist because pharma exists, like oxpeckers on rhinos. You will see companies ranging from tiny "mom-and-pop" operations in the family garage to monster companies employing thousands of people in regional offices around the globe. They will offer every kind of software "tool" you can imagine and some you cannot: electronic data capture programs, voice recognition, radiologic imaging digitalization, palm devices, statistical programs, and regulatory compliance programs, to name a few. They will offer their armies of workers to visit clinic sites anywhere in the world to educate local investigators, collect and check data on patients, and assist with Investigational Review Board requirements. They will offer high-level strategic consulting for regulatory strategies, reimbursement strategies, formulary management, communications plans, statisticians, medical writers, publishers, clinical trials registers and patient accruers, headhunters and recruiters, temp agencies, meetings organizers for doctors, nurses, or whoever. And at the DIA Exhibit Hall, you will also find public relations firms, legal experts, manufacturing experts, laboratory equipment, quality assurance, and quality control services.

If you wander the exhibit floor with Shubh, the first thing you will notice is that every few minutes, someone stops and calls out "Shubh!" The resulting reacquaintance is typically a series of big smiles, laughs, hugs, and nutshell summaries of life since they last

met. The family status is reviewed, as well as job pro-
gression. Calendars are checked to set dates to do
lunch, or breakfast, or drinks, or dinner. The years
have not diminished, but increased, the number and
warmth of these impromptu curbside chats.

The next thing you will observe on a walkabout
of the exhibit floor with Shubh is his banter, teasing,
and playful toying with inexperienced booth reps.
Occasionally, these reps will understand that they are
out of their league and will divert us to the director or
VP or whatever big shot they've got hanging out at
the center of the booth, to handle Shubh. The implicit
purpose of these five-minute forays is always to learn
as much as possible as fast as possible about each
other's businesses. And if the rep is a competitor, what
are his or her strengths and weaknesses? Or, is the
rep a potential partner with complementary services—
one that might be worth joining forces with?

The third thing you will notice in your DIA wander-
ings with Shubh is a pattern: most of the encounters
that he initiates are with attractive, smiling women. He
freely admits this when I tease him about it. He says,
"Why would I want to spend precious time with some
ugly, unhappy person when there are so many beautiful people in the world?"

Why, indeed, as he approaches his next victim
with his hand held out and his broad smile leading the
way. "How *aaare* you today?"

"Just fine, and you?" she twinkles.

"Wonderful … now that I've met *you!*"

8. "We Need to Teach Them How to Treat Us"

When I used to visit drug companies seeking project work, I was often asked this question: "*Who* do you work for?" They were actually asking me which group in pharma was the one that used our services and who was paying for our work. The answer wasn't simple. Any number of people or groups involved in developing or commercializing a product could be hiring and/ or paying MetaWorks. It usually boiled down to people in the areas of marketing, or in clinical Research and Development (R & D), or in regulatory affairs—and often all three. Information has lots of uses and users, but the ones who typically *paid* our bills were the marketers, because that's where nearly all the money is in pharma. It is debatable whether more pharma dollars are spent on marketing and sales vs. R & D, but from our perspective at MetaWorks, marketing was always the favored child, the banker for our project work. The dollars flowed from marketing wells, even when our clients were in R & D or regulatory affairs. Go figure.

The people we worked for had a fascinating and discontinuous mix of backgrounds, training, and goals, both personal and corporate. Our dream client, however, was someone with scientific training and experience, decision-making authority for the group, and a deep well of dollars to draw from. In reality, sometimes our client had only one of these distinctions, and sad to say, sometimes none. But all was not completely lost even in the latter instance, for if the client was a good communicator, or an effective delegator, much progress could be made. But when even those attributes were lacking, we might find ourselves in a really uncomfortable position as a consultant.

"Bad" clients are the ones who just don't "get it," never will, and don't know it, or don't care. MetaWorks had two such clients who fit this description, and these two are now and forever on our "blacklist." They are joined by a third individual—one who behaved unethically (in my book) or out of ignorance (in Shubh's kinder book). Regardless, in Shubh's words, when it comes to customers, "We need to teach them how to treat us." This oft-quoted Shubh-ism also applied to other service providers when *we* were the customers, as in the following typical travel scenario.

We rushed through a crazy morning at the office in order to get to the airport in time to check bags and go through endless security lines. Only after checking in were we told there was a two-hour delay, as the plane was stuck in Denver, or wherever, due to "weather." There were four of us on this trip, and we all followed Shubh to the Red Carpet Club, where he alone was a longtime member. Shubh apparently knew all the greeters behind the counter. They were sitting behind a sign on the counter that read "one guest per customer." The moment we crossed the Red Carpet threshold, one of the women called out,

"Long time no see, Mr. S! How've you been?"

Shubh smiled back. "It's great to be here, Laura ... I mean Linda," he said, as he got close enough to see the name tag. "My family and I would like to wait for our flight here today," he said, as he swept his arm at the three of us.

The smiling lady scrutinized his boarding

documents, glanced up suspiciously at the rest of us, and then held out her hand to gather our documents too. "Welcome, family! Come right in, all of you!"

Shubh congratulated her: "Now *you* know how to treat us right!"

Once we were finally on the plane, many long hours later, as the flight attendant slowly made her way down the aisle handing out ginger ale and Coke, Shubh raised his voice and asked her for free scotch for everyone.

"What?" she smiled, focusing in on him.

"Well, since you've kept us all waiting so long, it would be a nice gesture, wouldn't it? And if you don't have scotch, I'm sure whiskey will do."

"Well, sir, we don't usually do that when the delay is due to weather."

Shubh persisted, smiling, "But it'd be the *right* thing to do today, right?"

"Well … I'll ask the captain."

So she walked back to ask the captain and promptly returned, smiling. "I'm *very* happy to tell you we are offering free drinks on the house, for everyone!"

Immediately, a chorus of "thanks!" rang out, and the men in the seats around Shubh slapped high fives.

"Way to go!" and "You're the man!" resounded through the plane, accompanied by the cheerful clinks of a multitude of little Johnny Walker bottles.

Shubh just smiled, shaking his head slowly, saying to no one in particular, "We just need to *teach* them how to treat us!"

On our return trip, at the San Francisco Airport, we wound our way through the long ticketing line, waiting for the next available agent. Shubh scanned all the people sitting behind the counter, serving customers. "Which one do you think will be most moldable?"

I scanned them too.   The blond, middle-aged woman down the counter to our right got my nod. Shubh glanced her way and smiled. "Yes, I think you're right!"

But no sooner were the words out of his mouth than a customer from the first-class line rushed up to her. "Hmmm ... who else?"

"Does she have to be blond?" I asked.

"Preferably!" he smiled.

I spotted an agent with the appropriate "look," down the counter to our left.

"Okay, let's go for her."

It was our turn, and she was free, so we rushed up to her position. Shubh opened with a bright "Hello! How *aarrre* you today?"

"I'm just fine. How are you?"

"Well, my family and I are just fine, and we're hoping you will give us all first-class seats today."

She burst into a laugh.

"Your *family*, eh?"

She looked dubiously at all of us, three diverse-looking middle-aged women, backing him up at the counter. "I don't see *any* family resemblance here. Are you sure?"

"Oh, yes, and we'd like to sit near each other in your best seats."

She smiled broadly, as she looked over our picture IDs. "You all have different last names too. Are you sure you're all family?"

"Absolutely," Shubh beamed. We smiled stupidly. She mulled it over. "I know the *real* truth—they're your harem!"

This elicited a belly laugh from Shubh and uncomfortable squirms and shrugs from the rest of us.

She handed over all four boarding passes to Shubh. "Here, I know you'll want to keep these all together." She smiled.

In unison, we lunged forward to grab our own passes. "We'll take those separately, thanks! Really ... a harem? This joke's gone far enough, Shubh!"

As we walked toward the gate, we glanced at our boarding passes: free upgrades to business class all around.

"See? They *are* learning how to treat us," he said, as he fairly strutted toward the gate.

9. "There Ain't No Meta without No Data!"

Shubh and I were sitting in a corporate boardroom full of executives and senior managers, trying unsuccessfully to explain to them why it would be unwise to proceed with a meta-analysis, given the sorry state of their source data. We were trying to be diplomatic with regard to all the problems we could see in the useless studies they'd already wasted millions of dollars on. But ours was a message they just didn't want to hear. Finally, to our great relief, their own statistician, our hostess, ended the debate with this remark: "Guys, face the facts. What MetaWorks is trying to tell you is there ain't no meta without no data!"

Contrary to certain industry rumors, meta-analysis is not a way to produce something out of nothing. Meta-analysis cannot spin gold out of hay; rather, the truth is closer to "garbage in—garbage out." In order to do a good meta-analysis, you need good data. What does this mean?

The data we meta-analyze typically describe *groups* of people on clinical trials. Our unit of measure reflects the aggregate, or group, characteristics, such as the average age, or group response rate, as opposed to a *single* person's age or response status. Analyses of single patients on a clinical trial are the traditional statistician's job. Analyses of groups of patients on multiple clinical trials is the meta-analyst's job.

If we are going to analyze data from published clinical trials, we need to find all of the relevant trials and all of the relevant data from each of those trials, using predetermined criteria. This *a priori* approach

36

to selecting studies and data is a key feature of the research method that is a hallmark of our work: the systematic review method. Think about systematic reviews and meta-analyses using an oft-quoted but still handy analogy from the kitchen: making a stew. The flavor of the stew—or the results of the meta-analysis—depends upon the ingredients used and the method used to combine those ingredients. Experienced cooks can influence the outcome of their efforts by carefully choosing which ingredients to include and which to leave out, and whether to boil, simmer, or chill. So, too, can experienced meta-analysts influence an outcome.

While this fact might be useful to cooks in the kitchen, it can be hazardous when trying to use meta-analysis to find the truth. For if you can so easily influence the "truth" by *a priori* selection of which data to include, which to reject, and which statistics to use to combine data, the entire process is subject to substantial bias. In other words, I can influence the outcome of a meta-analysis by choosing to include certain studies that I believe might support my preconceived notions and by not including certain other studies that I happen to disagree with. To reduce the risk of this type of bias influencing your findings, you need to develop a protocol (i.e., a recipe) before starting the work. This plan should describe precisely what kinds of studies you seek and where you will find them, what data elements you will pull from each of those studies, and what kinds of analyses you will perform on the data that you find. This method of reviewing a complete body of clinical data with a view to synthesizing it reproducibly, explicitly, and in the most unbiased way possible is called a systematic review—the pivotal tool of clinical research synthesis.

Systematic reviews are superior to the traditional narrative reviews published in the medical literature, where a big name expert will typically discuss selected studies that support his or her opinions, whether stated or otherwise. That is, a typical narrative review reflects a process that is implicit, inherently biased, and certainly not reproducible—or defensible, for that matter. Systematic reviews are considered a huge improvement over traditional narrative reviews, and they have supplanted them almost completely in the medical literature since the time Chalmers and his colleagues first started promoting them. In pharma applications, the questions for clinical research synthesis are questions of efficacy or safety of a drug or treatment, by itself or in comparison with another drug or treatment.

The statistical method of meta-analysis is the most commonly used analytic technique to synthesize data quantitatively and reproducibly. But sometimes it is inappropriate to apply this tool to a particular dataset, such as when the ingredients are just too disparate, or too few, to combine meaningfully. That is, if you only had a single red-hot chili pepper, two apples, and powdered chocolate, you'd probably not try to combine them to make stew!

When a systematic review is performed in an academic setting, a team of people—senior investigators providing the "brains" and postgrads and other students providing the 'brawn"—will work for one to two years to complete it. It is not a trivial undertaking. MetaWorks' early claim of superiority over academics was speed. We assembled stable teams of experienced people who focused only on systematic reviews, working full-time, following standard operating procedures, and using a centralized relational database technology. In this way, we could cut the usual time for performance of a systematic review, with meta-analysis, from one year to three months. We could do it, and we could do it reproducibly, repeatedly. And we could do it even faster if we had to, as we'd demonstrated early on in our Pfizer calcium channel blocker project.

10. Using Information Better (in the Nick of Time)

A large pharmaceutical firm had a "me-too" drug for asthma. The drug had been FDA approved, and an imminent market launch was planned. The marketing group responsible for the launch believed that their "me-too" drug (drug "B") was actually superior to the first-to-market competitor (drug "A"). The group set aside many millions to perform a head-to-head comparison trial of its new drug B against the competitor's drug A. However, the statisticians involved in the clinical trial program for drug B had their doubts. They commissioned, from MetaWorks, a meta-analysis to support their opinion that a head-to-head trial of drugs B and A would not succeed. The primary objective of our review was, therefore, to determine the relative efficacy of these two drugs. Since no head-to-head comparison studies had ever been done, all published Randomized Controlled Trials (RCTs) of drug A vs. placebo and of drug B vs. placebo were sought. Unpublished trials were provided by the industry sponsor for its drug B, and the Summary Basis of Approval (SBA) for the competitor drug A was also obtained from the FDA.

Several typical asthma outcomes were assessed: forced expiratory volume in one second; peak expiratory flow rate, both morning and evening observations; and need for beta agonist rescue therapy. The efficacy estimate for each drug was established by using an effect size that compared each drug to placebo. The result of interest was the mean percent difference in the outcome (however measured) relative to placebo. All outcomes were assessed for all studies by drug type and over the full range of doses for which data were available, including the FDA-approved doses for each.

The effect sizes and corresponding 95 percent confidence intervals (i.e., the "wiggle room" around the estimate) all clearly overlapped for drug B and drug A at all doses of interest and for all outcomes noted above. The robustness of these results was tested in several additional sensitivity analyses. If only FDA-approved dosages of each drug, in adults only, were assessed, all results continued to favor each drug over placebo, and all 95 percent confidence intervals for each drug still overlapped almost completely.

Therefore, it was concluded that no matter what doses of drug A and B were assessed, or what outcome, or what patient population (adults or children), the treatment effects of drug A and B were nearly identical, with near complete overlap of their confidence bounds. A head-to-head study intended to show efficacy differences between these two drugs would be extremely unlikely to succeed. Estimated sample sizes required to narrow the confidence intervals sufficiently to eliminate overlap were particularly discouraging, in excess of 30,000 patients! With this best available evidence in hand, the sponsor made the correct decision to abort the trial before it ever started. Time and money were saved, and patients were spared participation in a useless study. Furthermore, the sponsor decided to pull the plug on the market launch of drug B, given its new, fully informed understanding that the costs of trying to beat the first-to-market competitor were not likely to be offset by sales revenues.

11. "We Do Data Right"

In early 1997, MetaWorks competed with over thirty groups around the country to win a much coveted designation as an Evidence-Based Practice Center (EPC) by the Agency for Health Care Policy and Research (AHCPR then, but now called the Agency for Healthcare Research and Quality, or AHRQ). Twelve EPCs were awarded five-year contracts to perform evidence reviews for the AHCPR on high-priority health care questions. MetaWorks was the only private sector, for-profit entity to win this contract. It wasn't the promise of a guaranteed amount of funded work that attracted us, but rather the clear statement to the world that MetaWorks had "passed mustard" (as Shubh said) with an independent and eminent third party, no less than a U.S. government agency. I was still trying to erase the ugly mental image of passing mustard, when Shubh crowed, "Now we can advertise like Boston Chicken!"

"How's that?"

"Because EPC says to the world, 'We do data right!' We do *chicken* right … we do *data* right! Get it?"

The EPC designation served notice to all that, even after losing Tom, MetaWorks still knew how to cook its chicken right.

Of course, the AHRQ projects were always a mixed blessing. On the upside, they gave our staff the chance to work closely with a client sector outside of our usual drug company roster. Namely, we got to work with the topic nominators on the projects funded by the AHRQ, which included Blue Cross Blue Shield, the Centers for Disease Control in Atlanta, Kaiser Permanente, and the

42

Social Security Administration. On the downside, the strain on our organization just to satisfy the enormous administrative requirements of these contracts was huge. I don't think we ever made a profit on a single one. But far worse, in the end, was seeing all our work end up in a useless, obsolete format—namely, three-inch-thick text documents destined to gather dust on library shelves, largely unread and unused. Like the Ark of the Covenant in the final scene of Indiana Jones, our reports would end up stored in some giant government warehouse, lost forever.

This occurred at a time when new information technology was exploding, and data was like a mighty Niagara; all we needed was a little creative application of that technology to really harness the power of the river. Like all EPCs, we dutifully produced one report after another. But the required formats for deliverables were passé, and the content was stale by the time our work was finally published by the government printing office. With the shelf life of medical information ever shortening, to wait eighteen months for publication was the equivalent of putting three-day-old bread on the bakery shelves.

Despite the obvious marketing advantages our EPC designation gave us, and the cross-pollination opportunities it afforded our scientific staff, we did not renew our AHRQ contract when it expired five years later. We could not overcome our extreme frustration in dealing with a large and plodding government bureaucracy and the unshakeable sense of futility that we felt, wondering if our government work made any real difference to anyone in health care.

12. "I Love Myself, and Something *Wonderful* Is Going to Happen to Me Today!"

"I love myself, and something *wonderful* is going to happen to me today!" Can you imagine saying this to a complete stranger? Before meeting Shubh, I would never have believed it could be done (1) with a straight face and (2) without sending people fleeing. The first time I heard Shubh coach a complete stranger with this mantra (I think we were in an elevator), I was mightily embarrassed and amazed that he didn't get smacked in the jaw. But no, his unwitting "student" just laughed and did not hesitate to repeat the mantra after him—as did countless others in our travels.

In particular, I'm reminded of a West Coast biotech company situated in a lush green campus-like setting in a tony suburb. In the main lobby of the main building, behind the reception desk, sat Esther, a fastidious, rather brittle-looking older woman who coolly greeted and handed out visitor passes to all who entered. Esther was the gatekeeper, and she was extremely efficient. She was also a great fan of Shubh's. He and I used to visit this company about once a month. We had lots of project work there, and it had such an active pipeline of products that it was ever a ripe prospect for new business.

On every visit, we'd arrive in the main lobby, and Esther would be there, prim and proper, stationed behind a long marble counter. Shubh's mission from day one was to teach Esther that we were not just "vendors," but rather, "friends." Within moments of our first visit, Shubh had asked Esther, "Do you like living in California?"

This simple question had opened a floodgate. We heard about her childhood on a farm in Indiana, her brief married happiness in Las Vegas, her lonely widowhood in the desert, and new beginnings in California. Esther had then continued to confide in Shubh that her day hadn't started out so well. She'd lost a hubcap on her way to work, she'd gotten a run in her stocking, some doctor calling the company had been rude to her on the phone, and her good friend in Building 22 was having a breast biopsy that day. Like a father confessor, Shubh listened to it all thoughtfully and solemnly, and then said, "All that, and it's only ten in the morning! Things are bound to improve as the day goes on, right?"

"Well ... I don't know."

He then said, "Esther, repeat this mantra after me: I love myself, and something *wonderful* is going to happen to me today."

She laughed nervously but then, without hesitation, intoned, "I *love* myself, and something wonderful is going to happen to me today." She smiled as she said it and added, "Hey! That felt *gooood!*"

"See, my friend? Say it often enough, and you will believe it. And if you believe it, it will happen! Trust me!"

"Oh, I do!"

"Then I want you to look at yourself every morning in the mirror and say it three times to yourself before you leave for work. Okay?"

"Okay!" she beamed.

That December, we were back at the same company. It was only a week until Christmas, and Shubh reminded me that we just couldn't show up without holiday gifts in hand, especially for Esther. My first reaction was that presents for all the admins would really add up, given that we dealt with so many different groups in project administration, research, marketing, and accounting—at least ten or twelve, I figured. Shubh stopped in his tracks and stared at me with a look of barely contained forbearance of my complete ignorance of business etiquette.

"Susan, you know it's the little people who matter most. It's the admin who will get the big cheese to return our phone call. She'll make sure our invoices get paid promptly. And she'll find appointment time on everybody's calendars for our meetings. We need to always be friends with the little people; we have to skid the grease!"

"Skid the grease? Or grease the skids?" I smiled.

"Aw … you know what I mean!"

Indeed I did, so I drove our red Cadillac rental to the mall before going over to the company. We found a very fancy chocolatier and ended up hauling out twelve very large boxes of expensive chocolates. When we arrived at our client's reception area with armloads of the beautifully wrapped stash, Shubh beamed at Esther, saying loudly, "Esther! Remember? I love myself, and something *wonderful* is going to happen to me today. Ho! Ho! Ho!"

Esther's jaw dropped in amazement as he handed her one of the boxes. "This is for you, Esther. Merry Christmas!"

Before she could answer, he asked her to help him deliver the others to all the administrative assistants and invoice clerks we worked with. "Here, I've got a list," he said, as he rummaged in his coat pocket.

"Wow! No one has ever been so thoughtful!" she effused.

Shubh smiled. "Well, you all deserve it, don't you?"

"You bet we do, but we don't usually get it!"

From that day forward, whenever Shubh and I returned to this company, upon entering the reception area, Esther would stand up with her arms outstretched in greeting and call out with a smile, "I *love* myself, and something *wonderful* is going to happen today! Come in, come in, come in!"

The crowd of vendors waiting in the lobby would glance up in unison, no doubt all wondering the same thing, "How does *that* guy get special treatment?"

13. Using Information Better (but Too Late)

A small East Coast biotech firm had funded several very encouraging Phase 1 and 2 studies, including a randomized trial, of its drug in the treatment of patients with metastatic kidney cancer. Based upon the favorable results of the randomized trial, a decision was made to undertake a pivotal trial for a regulatory submission. This pivotal trial was difficult to plan because the appropriate control regimen was highly debatable. Finally, after consulting not only the regulatory authorities, but also several internationally recognized opinion leaders, on the treatment of patients with metastatic kidney cancer, interferon alpha was chosen as the control arm treatment. This seemed to be a good choice at the time because it, like the experimental treatment, had relatively low toxicity and could be administered in an outpatient setting. The clinical experts confidently stated that, based upon their extensive off-label experience with interferon, the median survival for interferon-treated patients with metastatic disease would not exceed eight to nine months. Given the repeated demonstration in early trials of a median survival of at least fifteen months in patients receiving the company's experimental drug, the trial was designed to show an improvement in median survival from nine months in the control group to fifteen months in the experimental group. An FDA-experienced statistical consultant was also hired to assist with the trial design. Everything seemed to have been planned correctly.

Three years later, as the trial was finishing and the data were analyzed, the company was pleased to see that the experimental group had indeed achieved a fifteen-month median survival, exactly as predicted. However, the interferon control group had achieved a twelve-month median survival, considerably better than anticipated. The between-group difference in median survival was therefore not large enough to reach statistical significance given the sample size, which had been based upon an anticipated nine-month survival in the control group. In an attempt to understand what had happened, and with the hope of possibly showing that the interferon group outcome was a one-time aberration, the company asked MetaWorks to perform a systematic review of the literature on outcomes with interferon in metastatic kidney cancer.

This clearly showed that median survival with interferon could have been predicted to be 11.5 months, using only the literature that was available at the time the pivotal trial was planned, which was three years earlier. In studies that reported survival results for subgroups of interferon patients who most closely matched (by site and number of metastases, performance score, and prior nephrectomy) the patients in the pivotal trial control arm, the median survival was even higher, at 12.2 months.

This information could have been known at the time the company's pivotal trial was planned, had a systematic review of the literature been performed. The *JAMA* paper that Tom Chalmers and colleagues had published in 1992 had demonstrated how the opinions of experts often lag behind the evidence. Regrettably, this was but one more example.

The consequences of this failed trial were onerous. The patients on the study did reasonably well clinically and had probably not missed an opportunity to receive any other proven therapy. There were none that had been shown to prolong survival. However, these patients needlessly and trustingly donated their time and well-being to a failed study—a failure that might have been predicted, had a systematic review preceded the trial design. Furthermore, future patients will never have the opportunity to receive the company's experimental drug, which is very possibly useful in this condition. The company's drug will never be approved, let alone marketed, because there are no more funds for yet another trial. Several million dollars had been spent on the failed trial. The company had no cash reserves and was eventually sold. The entire program was ultimately consigned to oblivion.

14. "Wonderful! Now That I've Met *You!*"

The American Society of Clinical Oncologists (ASCO) is an annual pilgrimage for the MetaWorks business development group. Each day that we're at ASCO, Shubh schedules breakfast, lunch, and dinner meetings, with a few in-between, too, with old friends and clients. Nearly all of our corporate clients are also at this meeting every year, so it's a very convenient way to cultivate these crucial relationships. For Shubh, business development—life in general—is all about building relationships.

As at any of these annual mega-meetings, there is an enormous amount of behind-the-scenes hobnobbing among pharma researchers and product managers and the vendors servicing them. In fact, it is like two meetings running in parallel: the science meetings that all the doctors eagerly attend, and the business meetings that all the companies and vendors arrange.

We managed to have a pre-lunch meeting with one of our data providers, a database company, then went on to lunch with Chiron, had dinner with a MetaWorks clinical consultant, breakfast with Johnson & Johnson, lunch with Bristol Myers Squibb, and afternoon coffee with Abbott. The purpose of all these meetings was to discuss project ideas and proposals. Much was accomplished. Indigestion ensued. Shubh got by with frequent heavy doses of his personal supply of Pepsid AC.

We also sometimes manage to squeeze in a scientific session or two at these meetings. Late in the day, we hiked over to one of the dark and cavernous halls to hear a presentation that had been much hyped by the Genentech booth reps. We were supposed to hear about a new colorectal cancer treatment, and we'd been told that an extremely exciting breakthrough was going to be announced. Although the conference hall must hold thousands of people, it was standing-room-only when we finally arrived, five minutes into the presentation. The speaker's image was projected on huge TV screens suspended from the ceiling all around the hall, and his voice was booming in surround sound. We arrived just in time to hear the big news: the new drug had yielded a median survival advantage of 2.7 months, compared with patients who received the current standard of care.

"That's *it*?" I whispered to Shubh.

"Yup. *Incremental* improvement ..."

Then he added: "Last year's 'big breakthrough' has already flopped in the market."

However, the reporters and Wall Street analysts arrayed around the fringes of the room were clearly excited. Their cell phones were ringing, and some were bolting out the back doors to send their scoops back home.

Watching their exodus, I commented: "Isn't it a shame that everyone has such low expectations?"

In oncology drug development, a really small incremental improvement in a single study of a few dozen highly selected patients is enough to make headlines and double stock prices before the end of the day!

Shubh whispered, "Let's go. These poison pushers are killing me!"

We went to dinner with an industry consultant who pinch-hits for MetaWorks now and then, providing

PhD "bench strength" to our in-house scientific staff. Shubh took us to a restaurant at one of those trendy new "W" hotels. Although it was right on the lakeshore, with great views out over the water, "W" was a dark experience. The valet parking staff were all dressed like Neo in *The Matrix*. The "W" uniform is black turtlenecks, black trench coats, and sunglasses, even at dusk on a gloomy day. Inside the restaurant, it was dark—*very* dark. It seemed that the only light in the lobby bar was from a few tea candles scattered about on cocktail tables. My eyes did not adjust well, and I was stumbling forward while Shubh was excitedly hugging someone just ahead of us in the gloom. She—our hostess, it turned out—reciprocated. Having met her two weeks ago, while here on another Chicago visit, this was suddenly old home week for Shubh. And for her, too, it seemed.

Brittany beamed, as she strode forward to plant a kiss on his cheek, "How *aaarrre* you?"

"Wonderful, now that I've met you—again!" Shubh reciprocated with gusto. "I've brought my friends to experience your fabulous restaurant!"

"Well, I'm glad you did! It's so wonderful to see you again!"

"Do you have a great seat for us?"

"Of course! Right this way." She led us through the dark to a table only slightly better lit than the bar, near the window facing the lake.

As he took his seat, Shubh inquired, "Is my friend Charles here tonight to serve us?"

"No, I'm afraid Charles is off today. It's his birthday. But we'll take good care of you; don't you worry!"

She smiled, just as a slim, young man dressed all in black approached our table. "Good evening, sir."

"Oh, that's too bad," Shubh said. "Charles was outstanding!" Then he turned to the new arrival. "Young man, are you as good as Charles is?"

He didn't miss a beat. "You bet I am!"

"Well, I expect nothing less than the excellent service I had here last time with Charles."

"I'm sure you'll be pleased with your experience tonight, sir. My name is Jerome."

Shubh beamed. "Okay, Jerome! Then let's get started!"

And by this, he did *not* mean only the meal. At Shubh's prompting, Jerome unloaded a boatload of personal information over the next two hours. The off-beat story of young Jerome's life was served, for all of us to savor, in a series of snippets offered between courses. And his service was impeccable. Shubh provided career counseling throughout the evening. When it was time for us to leave, he handed Jerome his business card, with some final advice. "Contact me if you ever come to Boston. And stay in touch with your mother, young man. She always knows what's best for you!"

Before leaving Chicago, Shubh insisted upon giving me his personal tour of the University of Chicago campus. This was his first home after he arrived in America as a scared eighteen-year-old from a faraway land. For the first seven years after Shubh arrived here, he lived in the International House on campus. As we drove by the handsome neo-Gothic building, he recalled his first morning on campus so many years ago, when he was rudely blasted from a jet-lagged sleep, groggy and disoriented, by the booming voice of a woman twice his size, the college housekeeper, as she entered his room to clean it. Scared out of his wits, he couldn't remember where he was, let alone speak. He couldn't fathom who this intruder could be, blocking his doorway and yelling at him in a language he could not understand. He bolted from his bed, lunging for his clothes. It was many days later, after daily encounters with this frightful apparition, that he realized she was speaking English, but it was an inner-city variant that he never understood. With a little sigh of regret, he wistfully, but sincerely, concluded his story: "She took good care of me, but I was never able to communicate with that woman."

Later that day, as we returned our car to the airport rental lot, Shubh asked if someone would provide valet service to us, since we were running late, and he *was* a President's Club member, after all. The first two car check-in agents just scowled at this request and ignored us. But then, quite suddenly, a hard-faced man appeared at the driver's door and gruffly asked Shubh to move over. He would drive us to the United terminal at O'Hare.

As he clicked his seat belt, the driver muttered lowly, "How are you today, sir?"

"Wonderful! Now that I've met you!"

"Really?" he smiled and made eye contact with Shubh, who had slid into the front passenger seat.

"Sure! What's your name, my good man?"

"Henderson."

"Henderson. Is that your last name?"

"No, that's my first name. My last name is Gillespie."

Shubh repeated slowly: "Hen-der-son Gill-es-pie. That's a fine, important name."

"Yes, sir." And then he added, matter-of-factly: "And Dizzy Gillespie is my cousin."

"No! Really?"

"Yes, really. I saw him play a few times when I was a little boy, in New Orleans. He was pretty good."

"Sure, he was! And do you play a musical instrument?"

"Nah, not really. I tried trumpet but wasn't any good. I tried guitar, and I was better at that. I did play in a group for a while but not any more."

"I guess the good Lord gives us all different talents, doesn't he?"

"Yes, he does. I tried out basketball, too, but I wasn't tall enough. So now I work here. I like it here." He smiles at Shubh.

"Yup, you've got to find the right thing in life. And thank God we're all different, eh?"

"You betcha. You gotta follow what you're good at."

"Yes, you do!" And as we pull up to the curb, Shubh extends his hand for a handshake.

"Now thank you, my friend. You have a great evening."

"Yes, I will. And you too. It's been a pleasure." He is now beaming.

As we walk into the terminal, Shubh reminds me: "You never know who you're going to meet, do you? And they're always pretty interesting!"

15. Using Information Better (to Demonstrate

Class Effects—or Not)

A multinational pharmaceutical firm was planning a market launch of a me-too statin drug. While preregistration trials had proven efficacy in reducing cholesterol, there was no evidence yet existing that proved the drug's ability to impact important clinical outcomes in a beneficial way. In other words, there were no studies showing reduced mortality or heart attacks as a result of using the sponsor's statin, and it would take several years and millions of dollars of clinical trial expenses to complete such studies. However, there were several other statins on the market already, which had been studied for many more years than the sponsor's statin. These other statins had been studied in very large, multicenter trials of many years duration and had proven efficacy in terms of the mortality and heart attack outcomes that prescribing clinicians and formulary managers would demand. Therefore, the company wondered if it could jump on the coattails of these earlier statins in terms of these clinical outcomes, by demonstrating no differences among them for cholesterol lowering, and thus suggesting a "class effect" whereby all statins could be predicted to also have similar clinical effects upon treated populations.

MetaWorks performed a systematic review and meta-analysis of the world literature, describing these long-term clinical endpoints for the three already marketed statins. This meta-analysis showed convincingly that there were no apparent differences among the three statins studied, regardless of which clinical outcome was considered. Thereby, a class effect was supported. We decided to submit these results in a manuscript to a top-tier general medicine journal. Our manuscript was accepted for publication. The sponsor could then point to published support for its contention that all statins behaved similarly, in terms of clinical outcomes. Since its pricing strategy for its statin was designed to undercut the prices of the already marketed statins, this strategy was very helpful in gaining a decent market share of an already crowded but lucrative market.

Meta-analysis can also sometimes be helpful in showing where a class effect does not exist. An established pharmaceutical firm had in-licensed from an upstart biotech company a biologic agent to co-market for use as an anti-platelet agent in patients with acute coronary syndromes who were undergoing percutaneous coronary interventions, namely angioplasties or stent insertions. This first-to-market agent was soon facing stiff competition, however, from follow-on drugs which claimed to be similar in anti-platelet effect and, therefore, similar in clinical benefit. The competition was claiming a class effect that the sponsor had reason to doubt, based upon small, but potentially important, molecular differences among the agents. Therefore, a systematic review and meta-analysis was commissioned whereby MetaWorks collected data from all relevant published trials and then performed indirect comparisons of efficacy and safety of the three agents on the market.

At the time, indirect comparisons using meta-analysis were a leading-edge application of meta-analytic techniques. In essence, this work demonstrated that if no head-to-head trials existed for a direct comparison of competing agents, then indirect comparisons could sometimes be made that were statistically valid and clinically useful. MetaWorks was able to show that there was good reason to doubt the existence of a class effect in this case and that the sponsor's agent was demonstrably superior in terms of clinical outcomes when compared indirectly to the other two agents. This demonstration provided the sponsor with a strong argument to justify preferential prescribing of its agent, as well as formulary decisions about which of the three agents to list. In an important way, this early work heralded current trends in comparative effectiveness research.

16. "Let's Pray That She Is Looking Down on Us Today"

The trappings of success had their desired effect. The company's lush marble lobby was making me feel small, when Shubh suddenly intoned, "Let's pray that she is looking down on us today."

I looked around. "Who?"

"The Goddess of the universe, of course! Did you think God was a man?"

For Shubh, the all-powerful, all-knowing spirit of the universe is a "she." Why? Perhaps a female deity appeals to the iconoclast in him, and maybe also to the Hindu. Although a female deity is certainly at odds with the veiled misogyny of Christianity, which he'd embraced around the same time he dropped his vegetarianism, the Mother Goddess maintained a stubborn hold on him. Whenever we needed some extra good luck, he called upon her to "look down on us today." And, yes, she did look down on us that day. Marble-lobby, Inc., eventually became our very best client on the West Coast.

As a result, we visited that coast frequently, and we always rented a Cadillac. At first, it was a joke. In the northeast city where I grew up, Cadillacs were "ghetto" cars, driven by shady underworld characters. And while Cadillacs thus suited my low impression of Los Angeles, they did not at all suit my self-image. Yet Cadillac had the last laugh, as I became a convert. The big cars we rented were very comfortable and were also great for driving on LA's crowded freeways, floating and bobbing, cool and aloof, through the frenzied traffic. Since red is my favorite color, we always asked for, and usually got, a red Cadillac. For Shubh, the most important attribute of the Cadillac was that it gave us the *look* of Californian success. For him, this look was critical. There was no way we would show up at a prospective client's office in a little, shabby car. That would not suit Shubh's self-image. That would be almost as bad as admitting we'd stayed at a Holiday Inn Express—which we frequently did, of course.

Nevertheless, I still felt a little ridiculous behind the wheel of a Caddy. Yet I always insisted on driving, as would you, if you ever experienced the terror of riding with Shubh in the driver's seat. I think it may have something to do with his learning to drive in India's mayhem, but the toxic mix of a heavy foot, a cell phone, and no sense of direction that Shubh brought to the driver's seat was something you didn't want to experience twice as a helpless passenger. My own mantra for driving with Shubh was "once a passenger, always a driver." And I refused to let him sit in the backseat; he would have loved to pretend I was his chauffeur. So, sitting next to me in the front, he switched into his *Dragnet* routine. In his best Joe Friday voice, he launched a monologue, talking into a pretend police radio.

"At 10:27 a.m., my partner and I bid adios to Mrs. Chakrabarty at the Holiday Inn Express and drive north out of Manhattan Beach. Traffic is heavy but parts to let us through. Our destination? Company X, where, like all the best consultants, Susan will tell them again that they are fat, dumb, and happy. And they will love us for telling them so. It is a fact, and we always stick to the facts, just the facts, ma'am."

To make the most use of our time in California, we would visit as many clients as possible. This meant we'd often find ourselves cruising north from San Diego toward LA on Route 5 in our big red Cadillac. We always had to slow down at a checkpoint that was set up on the highway in the middle of nowhere, so that the immigration police could take a good look at us. The officers would wave most cars through but would stop the occasional car to look in the trunk or check papers of occupants. Whenever we approached this checkpoint, Shubh worried. He'd tighten his necktie and check his hair in the visor mirror.

"They might think I'm illegal. I do look a little like a Mexican, don't I?"

"Yeah, they'll haul *you* away in a heartbeat! But don't worry. I'll tell your wife where you are."

Needless to say, we always coasted right through, and he'd smile and wave vigorously at the officers. Then, breathing a sigh of relief, he'd say, "I guess they figure illegal Mexicans don't travel in red Cadillacs with blond lady chauffeurs!"

Continuing to head north, we'd eventually arrive at the heart of Orange County, near Irvine, where Shubh would point eagerly out his window, asking me this question: "Have you ever seen the Crystal Cathedral?"

"It's pretty hard to miss, Shubh!"

In fact, it's enormous, with blinding glassy surfaces jutting out at sharp modern angles, reflecting the intense California sunlight in all directions. As I recall, an enormous white cross adorns the roof. It looks like no church I've ever been to.

"Do you want to go visit it?"

"Not really."

"Have you ever heard of the Reverend Schuller?"

"No."

"Really?" he asked, with a look of mock shock. "You've *never* heard of Reverend Schuller?"

"Nope. Who's that?"

This was his invitation to tell me (yet again) about the many stirring sermons of the famous preacher, as well as his weekly TV show, *Hour of Power*.

"Ha! Ha! I can't believe he calls his show "Hour of Power"! Don't you think those guys are just charlatans? Just in it for the money? Like Jim and Tammy Bakker?"

"No way! Not the Reverend Schuller! He's really doing the work of the Lord. He inspires people. That's good, isn't it?"

"Well, maybe."

"You know, his son is also a preacher and will take over when Daddy retires." Then he'd smile and add, reading my mind: "I do agree it must be a very lucrative family business—not like MetaWorks! I wonder what she thinks of all this?"

"Yes, I wonder ..."

"Maybe we are in the wrong business!"

Then, after a long moment of silence as he scanned the horizon for a final glimpse of the glimmering church, he'd circle back. "C'mon, let's go see the Crystal Cathedral!"

17. Using Information Better (but Not Always)

The cardiac arrhythmia population in the United States is estimated at over two million people. Our pharmaceutical company client had a new anti-arrhythmic drug that was expected to be approved at the FDA within three months and was scheduled for a marketing launch three months after that. The company sought to support its marketing efforts by placing its clinical trial results in the context of what was *knowable* from the literature. It therefore commissioned MetaWorks to systematically map the treatment literature in atrial fibrillation. There were hundreds of studies published, but this was a case of "water, water everywhere, but not a drop to drink." Not many of these studies had the information the sponsor wanted. Specifically, our sponsor wanted to know the results of exercise tolerance tests in patients with atrial fibrillation, according to whether they were treated for rate control or for rhythm control. The sponsor also wanted to know which clinical outcomes (symptoms, activities of daily living, quality of life, and survival) were best supported by existing data in the atrial fibrillation literature, and in which areas its clinical program had, and might yet, fill information gaps for both prescribing clinicians and cardiology researchers. This was a perfect use of systematic review methods and a database-navigating tool such as the one we had built at MetaWorks.

We performed a systematic review of the atrial fibrillation literature, with distillation of results of studies of exercise testing as well as the other clinical outcomes of interest, into a hierarchical series of computerized evidence tables that could be delivered on a CD-ROM in which the various data elements of the various studies were readily sortable, searchable, filterable, and exportable. We called this type of study database "MetaHub," and we set it up, in this instance, according to type of exercise test, by type of treatment, by chronicity of disease, by etiology of disease, by geographic location, and by year of study. This permitted the company to use an evidence-linked communications plan in its marketing efforts, for both North America and Europe. The drug has subsequently been launched into the marketplace, and has done well, which is no surprise, given the intelligence and foresight demonstrated by its sponsors in seeking to root its value messages in tangible and immediately accessible, peer-reviewed evidence.

In a later example of smart corporate use of information, a savvy West Coast biotech firm anticipated launch of its recently approved breakthrough biologic for rheumatoid arthritis (RA). It recognized that this high-priced and difficult-to-administer agent would be entering a very crowded therapeutic landscape of well-established grandfather drugs. This upstart product would need to have convincing evidence of efficacy and safety to be accepted by specialists and patients. Head-to-head trials to demonstrate efficacy relative to standard therapy had not yet been completed except in a few narrow settings against only one or two other drugs. This would not be sufficiently convincing to achieve the type of accelerated market launch curve the company hoped for, and needed, to begin to recoup its enormous R&D investment.

Wisely, the company decision makers planned to

use only evidence-based information in its marketing plans. They approached MetaWorks to develop the evidence in the most rigorous, comprehensive, and unbiased way possible. We would perform a systematic review of hundreds of articles from the world literature, describing all treatments of rheumatoid arthritis. We would also seek an AHRQ EPC attribution for our work, which is, in effect, the data equivalent of the "Good Housekeeping Seal of Approval." This evidence would also be offered to professional organizations developing clinical practice guidelines. Lastly, the computerized study database resulting from our systematic review would be made available, not via CD-ROM as in our original offering, but via the Internet. It would permit frequent updates, including "hot off the press," peer-reviewed information on rheumatoid arthritis treatments.

When we had completed our work, we demonstrated this RA treatment database to a national professional society to consider using in its clinical practice guidelines development activities. They loved it, but the fact that a corporate sponsor was involved in funding it led them to decline using it. It had to be tainted, somehow, in their opinion. The professional society attitude that corporate monies *must* taint systematic reviews only serves to create serious information inequities in health care. Such imbalances put ill-informed consumers, be they patients or providers, at the mercy of extremely well-informed sellers of new products. Unfortunately, this situation continues to this day.

The sponsor found numerous uses for this

information and continued to fund updates to the evidence base from our shop at regular and frequent intervals. They used this information to develop new clinical study hypotheses, to contextualize study results, for safety signal exploration in pharmacovigilance, as well as in marketing communications. The company's breakthrough product has gone on to achieve blockbuster status. To my everlasting disappointment, however, our Internet database concept has never been widely adopted in health care. Perhaps, with different funding, it might have succeeded? But funding from where? Until that question is answered, or someone develops a less expensive way to synthesize vast quantities of ever-evolving clinical data for the masses, the information inequities between the medical-industrial complex and health care consumers—between seller and buyer—will continue.

18. "You Can Doooo It!"

BWI Airport, Avis counter, 10:30 p.m. We've just arrived and need a car to get to an FDA meeting in the morning. As usual, Shubh has an advance reservation, and, as usual, Preferred Status. This is supposed to mean that we just pick up our rental agreement at the counter, find our waiting car in the lot, and drive away. But it rarely works out that way with Shubh.

On this night, we pick up our agreement, walk to the designated parking spot, and find a grey Buick LeSabre waiting for us. Shubh's face immediately clouds over. "Susan, we can't accept this. Let's go get a Cadillac. They need to do better than this donkey!"

"I'm okay with the Buick, really, Shubh. It's not like we're in LA and need a Cadillac or anything."

"Well, I think they should give us a Cadillac anyway!"

So we march back to the Avis center office. A faintly scowling man built like a refrigerator is sitting at a computer behind the counter. His body language says *do not disturb*!

Shubh forges ahead, lasering in on his name tag.

"Hello, Michael, my good man. My name is Shubh, I'm a Preferred member, and you're supposed to have a car for me tonight."

Michael never looks up from his typing.

"Yes, sir. Your car is out in the lot, in parking spot number 32."

"No, I don't want that car. You don't expect me to drive a Buick, do you? I think you should give me something better. Don't you have any Cadillacs?"

Michael, finally looking up, says, "I don't think so.

The LeSabre is a very good car, sir. It's the same class of car as a Cadillac."

"Ha! Now you don't really believe that, do you? Of course, it's not. I think you should get me a Cadillac. My friend here (pointing to me) will only drive Cadillacs. She is a doctor, a very important person, and you don't expect us to drive around in that lousy Buick, do you?"

Mortified, I'm ducking behind Shubh, while Michael sizes us both up. "Well ... no, I guess not, but I really don't have a Cadillac I can give you tonight."

"Yes, you do! Yes, you can! Look right over there! I've found one for you!" he crows triumphantly, pointing to spot number fourteen. "Now, it's not red, like we usually get, but we'll take it, even though it's silver."

Michael is now shaking his head back and forth, breaking into a wide smile.

Shubh smiles too.

"Come on, brother! You *know* that car's available. You *can* do the right thing and give it to me. You can make two very happy Avis customers! You've got the power! You can *doooo* it!"

Michael, to my amazement, suddenly acquiesces, saying softly: "Sure ... okay."

Shubh slides the Buick rental agreement back across the counter to him. Michael fidgets with some papers and hands out a new rental agreement to us.

"Spot number fourteen, sir. Enjoy it!"

"We *sure* will! Thank you *verrrry* much! You are going to go far, Michael. You have a wonderful evening now, you hear?"

So we drove happily away in our silver Cadillac,

heading unwittingly to Shubh's next motivational session at the Days Inn in Silver Spring, Maryland. It took
awhile to find it, and it was nearly midnight when we
arrived. The thick Plexiglas separating us from the
front desk receptionist should have been an instant
giveaway as to the caliber of the place.

Shubh joked and smiled at her, pointing to the
glass: "Is it bulletproof? Should we be afraid?"

But the young woman on the other side just glared
silently as she proceeded to check us in. Shubh passed
his credit card to her via the little swivel drawer in the
Plexiglas barrier, just as a highly muscled young man,
practically oozing testosterone, sauntered into the
lobby from the dark parking lot out front. He planted
himself right next to us at the glass and proceeded to
glower unblinkingly at Shubh. The surly front desk girl
shouted out our room numbers, as she placed the card
and our keys in the pass-through. Now we started to
feel uncomfortable, seeing as this rude young man had
clearly heard which rooms we'd be going to. Shubh
shot her a look of intense disapproval and then turned
to me.

"Do you want to just leave now?"

I was reluctant, because I was too tired to go
searching for another hotel late at night in this dark
and seemingly unsavory neighborhood. I just shook
my head.

"No, no ... this will be okay once we get to our
rooms. Let's stay."

So we picked up our bags and detoured around
the young man, who never budged.

But then, we couldn't find our rooms. The numbers

didn't run in any apparent order in the upstairs corridors, which, by the way, were littered with debris
and chips of paint falling off the cinder block walls. I'd
never stayed in such a decrepit-looking hotel, even in
my poor student days when I was hitchhiking on five
dollars a day through Europe. After ten minutes of
wandering around in the dim silent corridors, even after
backtracking to the lobby and starting over again—the
young man was now ominously gone, and the receptionist had disappeared too—we still could not find our
rooms.

"Hmmm. Are you sure you want to stay here?"

I shrugged but was indeed losing hope.

"Okay, let's try one more time."

So off we went again, but still we could not find our
rooms. When we found our way back to the lobby a
third time, Shubh turned to me and said, "I really think
we should go someplace else; shall we?"

This time, I didn't disagree.

By now, the receptionist was back at her post.
Shubh told her we had changed our minds and did
not want to stay. He asked her to void our credit card
imprints. She said she could not do that with less than
twenty-four hours notice, so he pointed to a sign right
in the window in front her, of which she was apparently
unaware. He read it aloud to her.

"It says here 'If any room does not pass the customer's inspection, the customer is not required to
accept it.' Well, we do not want to accept our rooms."

He didn't add that we never actually found our
rooms. That was immaterial at this point. Shubh

asked her again (three times, in fact) to void our bill, but each time she just shook her head.

"No, I cannot do that."

Shubh, in turn, and with ever increasing force, replied each time: "Yes ... you ...can!"

This debate was turning into a futile shouting match, which, in this neighborhood, might have deteriorated into an encounter with her scary friend, who was still nowhere to be seen. I headed for the door, hoping to draw Shubh away from the confrontation. But then suddenly, with complete poker face, she voided the bill and with a flourish, passed it back through the glass. She stared defiantly at Shubh, waiting for his angry retort. But he just smiled sweetly and said quietly, "You see? You can dooo it! I *knew* you could. Remember that, young lady, in everything you do. It's not your aptitude but your attitude that determines your altitude!"

For the first time that night, she smiled. He laughed and called out to her, as we hauled our luggage back outside, "Thank you, my friend, and have a good night!"

As we speed-walked past the young man, who was now standing in the parking lot watching us, Shubh nodded in his direction and smiled, "Good night, my friend."

And to my surprise, the young man smiled back. "And a pleasant evening to you too, sir!"

At that moment, I realized I may have misjudged this guy. Instead of planning evil deeds, he was actually guarding the receptionist from unruly customers like us!

So onward into the night we drove, not sure where exactly we were going, except in the general direction of Chevy Chase. We drove through a dark and sleeping suburban landscape until we spotted our next lodging candidate, a Holiday Inn. This place looked better than the last, except for the creepy underground parking lot. Our big silver steed took up two parking spots, but hey, it was late, and there was obviously not a big demand for parking spots in the cavernous and nearly empty lot. Shubh looked around vigilantly as our steps echoed in the subterranean murk, looking for a way back up to the surface and the hotel lobby. He grumbled, "Wow, we've been pushed to the back of the bus all night, haven't we?"

And then he added more brightly: "But we need to be more like Rosa Parks! She's my hero."

When we eventually emerged from the hotel underworld and located the lobby, we encountered three handsomely dressed foreign trainees working the reception desk, each wearing a little name tag displaying his name and home country. Without a common language among them, the three worked together ineptly but with great flair, attempting to check in a Japanese man who was as English-challenged as they were. At another time, another place, this Mad Hatter's tea party might have been amusing but not now. Only when the night manager came out from a room behind the desk was the check-in process expedited.

Finally, we had our keys, and we dragged our bags off to our rooms. Shubh, ever chivalrous, would typically accompany me to my hotel room at check-in to be sure it was satisfactory. Lo and behold, the dead-bolt lock to my room was broken. When he saw it, he said, "Come with me. You take my room. Then I'll go back down to the lobby to get another one for myself."

As our luck would have it that night, Shubh's door had neither a working handle lock nor a dead bolt—the door just pushed open from the corridor.

So back to the lobby we both went.

The trainees smiled quizzically. "Yes. Hi. You need something? Rooms okay?"

"No, rooms not okay! The doors don't lock. My door doesn't even latch shut!"

"What? Doors don't lock?" the trio echoed. They stared incredulously at each other.

"C'mon, guys. Give us new rooms. You can *doooo* it."

No one made a move.

"Get me the manager," Shubh growled.

"One moment, please," they said in unison, and they all disappeared into the manager's room behind the reception desk.

Finally, after aiming some angry barbs at the hapless night manager, with his nervous trainees taking it all in from a safe distance behind him, we had our keys for new rooms. Shubh muttered, "Well, if they can't do it, we can!" So back upstairs we trudged, and this time, all was satisfactory—until about 2:00 a.m.

I was just falling asleep when the fire alarm sounded. I stumbled up and scanned the fire instructions on the door, which seemed much too drastic to actually follow in the middle of a freezing winter night. I tried calling the front desk, but there was no answer. And then the hotel operator—also no answer. The awful high decibel alarm continued. Over the ringing, I heard doors opening and voices in the hallway, so I peeked out. There were several sleepy-eyed people leaning their heads out their doors, looking up and down the corridor, all wondering the same thing: *What should we do?* Suddenly, a very large black woman wearing a bright pink robe and curlers under a plastic kerchief came stomping down the center of the hall, announcing in a loud no-nonsense voice, "C'mon everybody. We're going down the stairs. We're going down the stairs!"

This was all the persuasion I needed. I hastily piled on several layers of clothing and my overcoat over my pajamas, grabbed my room key, and headed out into the hallway. I saw Shubh farther down the hall, looking around groggily. I waved and joined him, and we followed the strangely silent crowd down nine flights of stairs. At the bottom, we were greeted by the din of sirens and engines and people shouting directions to us to hurry up and get out into the parking lot.

There we huddled, freezing and grumbling, shivering in the dark for another forty-five minutes, waiting for the firemen to give the all-clear. Finally, they let us back into the lobby at 3:00 a.m., and then it was sheer pandemonium as the reception desk trainees and hotel guests sparred about room keys left behind in the confusion of our evacuation. Luckily, both Shubh and I had had the presence of mind to bring our keys, so we escaped a continuance of the evening's many aggravations.

Thus concluded another long night of business travel, another journey where Shubh refused to accept what he considered sub-par treatment. And he did it by empowering unmotivated strangers to change their attitudes, to do their jobs better. Unfortunately, we didn't have similar success at our FDA meeting the next day. Despite our best efforts at extolling the wonders and beauties of using meta-analyses for noninferiority trial designs, the meeting fell flat. Blame it on our sleep-deprived performance, or an audience long hardened to overtures like ours, but this was one time we just could not *dooooo* it.

19. Using Information Better

(to Avoid a Clinical Trial)

An international pharmaceutical firm had FDA approval to market its acid-busting proton pump inhibitor to treat duodenal ulcer. Now it wished to extend the label to include an indication in gastric ulcer. This should have been straightforward, since they had several well-designed positive trials already completed. However, to satisfy the usual FDA requirements for "two adequate and well controlled trials," at least two of these trials would have be able to withstand an FDA audit, a point-by-point verification of each data element collected on each patient's case report form. The full paperwork documentation of the process used in each study would also have to be reviewed, if, in fact, it existed in the FDA required format.

The problem was that most of the sponsor's relevant trials had been completed in foreign countries, primarily Japan and Germany. The principal investigators and clinical study sites were not fully willing, and/or able, to comply with these FDA audit requirements. The corporate sponsor, therefore, asked MetaWorks to meta-analyze the data from all these trials together. They would then submit the analysis to the agency, along with the auditable data from the one American trial in the set.

MetaWorks obtained datasets from the sponsor's trials, and performed a meta-analysis of individual patient data, which is widely considered to be the strongest data type for meta-analysis. This permitted not only a demonstration of efficacy and safety but

also an exploration of best doses and dosing schedules. This meta-analysis was submitted to the FDA,
and along with the sponsor's single auditable trial data,
was the basis for eventual approval. The FDA review-
ers requested a copy of the meta-analysis database,
as well as the SAS programs used by our statisticians.
MetaWorks provided these, and the agency review-
ers took the data for a "test drive." They found the
results sufficiently convincing to grant the approval to
market the drug in the new indication of gastric ulcer.
MetaWorks' meta-analysis results are now included
on the product label.

This successful strategy, in effect, saved the sponsor from having to run yet another U.S.-based study,
which translates to millions of dollars saved in clinical
R & D costs and additional millions gained in getting to
market years earlier than would have been otherwise
possible. It also resulted in sparing more patients
from participating in a study that, in reality, was just
not necessary.

20. "Are We Fish or Fowl?"

Early on, we heard through a friend in an Asian-focused clinical research organization (CRO) that Singapore might be a good source of investment money. The government of that island state hoped to attract new "high technology" business to its shores, and was offering five-million-dollar grants, not loans, to qualifying companies. We thought it'd be a real kick to have an office in Singapore, with MetaWorkers working round the clock on both sides of the globe. And we could use the money to build MetaHub, our repository of data from systematic reviews. This data warehouse was going to be key to our future success, which, we hoped, hinged less on our consulting business and more on our producing a variety of information products for a variety of customers in health care. This identity confusion plagued us for years. We couldn't decide if we were fish or fowl, to use Shubh's analogy. Were we a consultancy or an information product company? Eventually, the market told us. We were definitely fish who should forget about flying. But that reality only sunk in later, years after our first pilgrimage to Singapore in search of transformation.

So we flew six hours to San Francisco, then another twelve to Hong Kong. While our CFO and I tried in vain to sleep in our economy seats, Shubh paced the aisles, happily chatting with every flight attendant he encountered. This was before 9/11, and he was permitted to loiter in the galley with "the girls," snacking, chatting, and laughing. Only once do I recall that he sat down and, in his typical fashion, closed his eyes and fell immediately into a deep sleep. After two hours, though, he was up again, pacing. By the time we landed in Hong Kong, I was stiff and groggy, but Shubh was in fine fiddle. But as we were jostled by pushy crowds of unsmiling people in the Hong Kong airport, his mood suddenly soured. He growled about the excessive rudeness of Hong Kong Chinese. These people were clearly immune to his smiles and friendly gestures. We stayed at that airport just long enough to brush our teeth in the restrooms, and then we climbed back onto another plane and headed down the Vietnamese coast to Singapore.

By the time we landed, I was in zombie mode. Shubh, however, was once again, after three more hours of partying in the galley, chipper and bright. We taxied to our hotel, where showers and a wonderful breakfast concoction of nasi goreng revived me and further energized Shubh. We then set out to meet our first potential alliance partners: a diverse assortment of academics, government officials, and corporate types.

This trip, with its busy schedule of meetings, was arranged for us by a friend of a friend—a well-connected Hong Kong native who'd been educated in London and had lived in Texas, but now worked deals as a local intermediary for businesses like ours with the government of Singapore. This fellow personally shepherded us from glitzy new building to glitzy new building. From inside Singapore's skyscrapers, the city felt just like New York or LA, except, of course, that the population was more homogenous, and nearly all were shorter than Shubh, which he enjoyed immensely.

That night, our host took us to his club. He

explained that, in Singapore, the only evening enter-
tainment to be had is that which you arrange privately.
The government is very strict about after-hours activities. Our travel books warned us that you could even
be arrested (up to one year in jail) for bringing chewing
gum into the country! Our host explained that everyone belonged to clubs, and he was obviously proud of
the fact that he belonged to the original British club on
the island.

And what a bastion of British culture it was. As
we moved from the hot and crowded sidewalk into
the cool, dark enclave, we also crossed time zones
and continents. As our eyes adjusted, we could see
that we stood in a lobby with mahogany wall panels
adorned with portraits of staid English matrons and
uniformed gentlemen, looming large above over-
stuffed chairs and potted palms. Our host led us
through the lobby into a perfect English pub, complete with India Pale Ale and Guinness on tap, and we
heard only English spoken, and only in stiff-upper-lip
British accents.

Shubh, like a chameleon, immediately started
speaking with a British accent too. Throughout the
evening, Shubh never broke his new accent. He
seemed to be unaware he was doing it, and no one
seemed to notice but me. I figured that Shubh, in his
eagerness to relate well with everyone, was just trying
to fit in. He never let up until we were alone in the taxi
after dinner, heading back to our hotel. I pointed out
to him that he was now speaking with an American
accent, after speaking British English all night. He
gave me a look of pure shock. "I am? I did?"

"Didn't you realize you were speaking with a British accent all evening?"

"No, I didn't!"

"Well, you did, but now you're back to basic American."

"Gee, I hope our host didn't notice," he said, looking truly contrite.

The next morning, we all regrouped for our next investor meeting. As Shubh drifted ahead of us on the sidewalk, our host leaned in to my ear and whispered, "Was Shubh making fun of me last night?"

I stopped walking and looked at him. "What do you mean?"

"I mean, his British accent—which I notice is gone today. Was he mimicking me?"

I fumbled for an explanation and tried to suggest that it was not *conscious* mimicry, in my opinion. I tried to explain that I'd seen Shubh switch into Italian and Spanish accents, as well as local accents in New York, New Jersey, and the American South. It happened wherever we traveled; if there was a strong local accent, you could count on Shubh echoing it faithfully. This was all true, but our host looked skeptical as he nodded his head. We caught up with Shubh, who smiled brightly and asked "I say, old chap, lovely morning, what?" in his most faithful British accent.

The Singapore money never materialized, but I doubt it was a problem of accents. Rather, Singapore was just too far away from Boston, in so many ways. Their long and evolving list of objections, requests, and requirements (although none that involved gum chewing!) was just too onerous to satisfy. Maybe they could see that we were only fish who wanted to fly. We probably should have realized this before we ever stepped onto a plane headed for Singapore, but sometimes the most obvious lessons need to be learned the hard way.

21. "Never Take Money When You *Need* It!"

Despite our Singapore failure, our business yielded a healthy and growing profit in the first few years, even enough to surprise our employees with year-end bonuses. In retrospect, it's clear that these bonuses were probably too generous, and like so many other decisions we made in those early days, quite unwise. We should have been banking our cash for a rainy day. For when it rained, it poured.

We had overhired in production but underhired in sales. Our head count had swelled to thirty-five, which was way too many, in retrospect, considering our revenues at the time. Cash flow turned persistently negative. We couldn't make payroll without resorting to personal credit cards, bank loans (with our homes as collateral), and loans from sympathetic family members. Furthermore, rather than patiently wait until we had the money to fund development of our data warehouse (MetaHub), we jumped the gun, incurring huge programming expenses with a software development company. We fully intended to pay them what we owed, a little each month, as our profits rolled in.

But one day, out of the blue, they demanded payment of our entire balance in full, immediately. We couldn't satisfy them. So they froze our bank accounts. Our lawyers jumped into action. But until we could persuade a judge to counter their preemptive strike, we had no choice but to try to find other quick money—and fast. We had rent and payroll to pay.

Needless to say, this is the worst possible position to negotiate any deal from, particularly with moneymen who are eager to take full advantage of your plight. It

84

is a very humbling experience, but one you will endure if your company survival is at stake. Our saviors were two interesting specimens from the venture capital jungle. These VCs provided the fast cash we needed to stay alive. But it came with truly onerous terms. We lost ownership of half our company in exchange for their investments. And they had little interest in our mission. They seemed interested in only one thing: a quick turnaround of several multiples on their money. And they were not happy to be "patient money." They had neither the interest nor the ability to help us gain clients or useful connections. After their bailout cash infusion, they made it clear they were unwilling to provide any additional funds for growth. To be fair, I guess our behavior hadn't entirely merited the level of enthusiasm or trust we had hoped for.

We knew it was a terrible trade-off, but we believed it was a life-or-death decision, so we chose life. Our forced coexistence with the VCs had a profoundly demoralizing effect upon senior management. But whenever one of us complained, Shubh would remind us that all entrepreneurs face huge hardships to keep a company alive if financing is not properly planned. He would argue that VCs can indeed be fair minded if their expectations are properly managed. He said we were like the toad in one of his favorite fables.

"You know the story of the toad who desperately needed to get across the river but couldn't swim, so he hitched a ride on the back of a water snake?"

"No."

"The snake smiled and promised the wary little toad that he would not harm him, so the toad trusted the snake and climbed aboard. When they were half way across the river, the snake flipped the toad into the air and sunk his formidable fangs into him. As the snake prepared to swallow him whole, the poor toad gasped, 'But you said you wouldn't hurt me!'"

"The snake smiled and replied, 'Yes, but you should have known I just can't help myself. A snake *never* loses his fangs.'"

And then Shubh would stab the air while pronouncing the moral of the story: "Never *ever* take money when you *need* it!"

22. "We're Living in the Taj Mahal!"

Our new VCs insisted on a new CEO—*their* man. In a matter of days, our embattled CEO unhappily departed, and their CEO arrived. This did not go over well with any of us, but least of all Shubh, for our new CEO was also a transplanted Brit. Although the British were no longer ruling India when he was growing up there, they had left behind a legacy: Pakistan. In creating Pakistan, they had authorized a national boundary line to be drawn straight through the heart of his family's estate. With the birth of Pakistan came hometown mayhem, and the death of his family fortune. So Shubh blamed the entire British Empire. Perhaps it was no surprise, therefore, that his gut-level dislike of the British colonizers in India carried over to the Brit who now colonized MetaWorks. Whether he realized it or not, our new CEO had stepped into a world of varied resentments when he stepped into MetaWorks. And regardless of the fairness, or lack thereof, of judging an individual on the basis of perceived national character traits, Shubh would sneer "the Brits are *goooood* at running companies … into the ground!"

In his opinion, they had a knack for corporate screw-ups, and then, like in India, they'd typically duck responsibility for the mess. He'd point to one of our West Coast data partners as a case in point. This company installed electronic medical records in doctors' offices and maintained a large data warehouse that MetaWorks could use as a data source for certain analyses. Their British CEO (also installed by investors) had spent their entire cash reserve of $12 million in the first twelve months. And there was nothing to show for it. Only after the company had blown through all its cash (on expensive new hires, first-class travel, and limousines, as far as we could see) was the Brit finally given the boot. The founder had to step back in, from his too-short retirement, to make the necessary and Draconian expense reductions necessary for survival. He had to fire over half of the employees the Brit had just hired.

Despite observing this sad scenario play out from afar, I was still not convinced that this British hang-up of Shubh's was anything we should take seriously. We had no choice anyway, as he who pays the piper calls the tune, and our VCs had paid the piper for us and hired a Brit to be our new boss. Our new CEO began by immediately moving us to a higher rent and (relatively) luxurious brass and mahogany office. Shubh shook his head in disapproval, and hung a three foot wide photograph of the Taj Mahal on his office wall. While I laughed, he ruefully said, "Well, we're living in the Taj Mahal now, aren't we?" It was twice the space we needed and opulent in comparison to the office we were leaving (forced out by Boston's never-ending tunneling project, the 'Big Dig'). Despite our elegant new surroundings, our new CEO insisted that all serious discussions with his senior staff would happen off-site, preferably in a place where food was served. Suddenly all our meetings were accompanied by coffee, drinks, lunch, breakfast, dinner—you name it. Meetings no longer took place in the Taj; was he afraid it was bugged? And at these meetings, which were numerous, no matter what we discussed, no matter how mundane, our new CEO treated it all as "top secret." He made us swear not to tell any others in the company what we discussed, no matter how innocuous the topic was. We were used to working in a completely open, "all for one and one for all" environment, so this secrecy fetish just felt wrong.

And to add insult to injury, if regular staff meetings at the Taj were attended by three or more people, our CEO invariably sat as far away from the group as he could; he was usually seated at the other end of the long conference table, not participating in the discussion, but furiously, silently, taking notes on a big yellow legal pad. Subsequently, he'd personally type it up (the material was too "sensitive" for his secretary to do this) and circulate pages and pages of near-verbatim transcript, asking for review and edits—as if anyone of us had time, or interest, in reviewing his notes! Let's just say they were promptly filed under "T"– (for trash). Soon, everyone started making excuses to avoid accepting his meeting requests, and it wasn't long thereafter before the organization was operating as if our CEO didn't exist at all.

Shubh, however, had near daily run-ins with him. For instance, to boost revenues, the new CEO insisted that we just raise our already-high prices 20 percent across the board, in one fell swoop. Shubh was livid, but complied. Thereafter, we lost bid after bid (on the basis of price), until we decided, in desperation, to just roll our prices back again, without discussing it with the CEO.

In the meantime, in the eight months since this CEO had been placed at the helm of the good ship MetaWorks, our expenses had risen out of control.

We had run aground, with an obscene and growing negative variance in our budget. Our CEO wasn't distressed by this, however. He would just ask the VCs on our Board for more money (and thus give them even greater control of our futures). In fact, he insisted that our ever-growing deficit was a good thing, of great value as a tax write-off to any future acquiring company. We responded to his cheerful plan by engineering a mutiny to get rid of him before it was too late.

At our next Board meeting, this CEO, as expected, asked our VCs to pump in yet more money—a *lot* of money. As they lifted their jaws off the conference table, I presented them with a simple alternative: either kill the company, or remove the new CEO and let us run it ourselves as a triumvirate, namely me, Shubh, and our "Rock of Gibraltar" in Operations, Janet. We would make a go of it without any new cash infusion. And so it happened.

23. "Shuuuubh...Shuuuubh...Shuuuubh"

From that day forward, Shubh-isms flourished at MetaWorks like never before. I served as president for the first post-Brit year. Janet continued to valiantly "herd the cats" in her role as VP Operations, and Shubh kept "feeding the hopper" as VP Marketing and Business Development. Time and again, to make payroll and pay rent, we had to borrow money against our accounts receivable. Our savior lender was my brother-in-law, since no bank would have us. It was a struggle, but Shubh kept us laughing. He and Janet and I called ourselves the SWAT Team, while our staff called us the Power Trio (and possibly a lot of other things we never heard about!). Although it was tougher than ever to make ends meet, it was a different kind of demand, the kind you can control, as opposed to the kind you cannot. Tom once said the only difference between pressure and stress was that you were in control with the former but not the latter. This was pressure, not stress.

With the Brit gone, Shubh acted like a huge weight had been lifted off his shoulders. He charged ahead with renewed energy to boost new bookings, which were our lifeblood. Eventually, we were able to pay off our debts and consistently keep our heads above water. After a year, I gladly moved aside, returning to my former role as Chief Science Officer, when Shubh agreed to take the president's position in our triumvirate.

Miraculously, he was then able to secure a banker who was willing to give us affordable credit. What a relief that was! Without a banker, we'd been walking a high wire without a safety net. Gingerly, we started to hire the expertise necessary for growth. We were then able to win another multi-year government contract with the National Institute of Child Health and Human Development (NICHD) to assess the evidence regarding efficacy and safety of prescription drugs in children, under the Best Pharmaceuticals for Children Act (BPCA). This was a wonderful restart for us. When it came time for our monthly all-staff meetings, Shubh would seize the office intercom and, with not a little self-mockery, mimic Colonel Klink, the clueless camp commandant on *Hogan's Heroes*.

"Attention! Attention! Attention! All employees report at once to the boardroom! All employees report to the boardroom at once!"

To start these meetings, he'd play the theme song to *Mission Impossible* on my tinny-sounding portable tape player. To end the meetings, he'd lead the group in a meditative exercise, exhorting everyone to close their eyes and intone, not "Om," but "Shuuuubh ... Shuuuuubh ... Shuuuubh." This "meditation" invariably had the desired effect: belly laughs all around. We were having fun again after a long and painful dry spell.

24. "If You Keep On Doing What You're Doing, You'll Keep On Getting What You're Getting!"

Over the next few years at MetaWorks, we faced a daily struggle to preserve our scientific integrity *and* still make a profit. We steered very carefully between our particular Scylla and Charybdis: purism and pandering. If we were completely inflexible regarding our meta-analysis methods, for instance, we might lose a project and a client. Just as importantly, if too inflexible, we might lose an opportunity to push the envelope on a statistical method or application, and thus advance the field. On the other hand, if we caved in to every silliness that corporate clients wanted, we'd be pandering and guilty of bad science. With the passage of time, it became easier to hold our mid-channel course, because the environment changed, and our reputation for good science grew. The principles and practices of evidence-based medicine gained real traction in the industry, and our growing reputation for excellence gave us more gravitas to face down untenable requests from clients.

But along the way, our business ebbed and flowed, from season to season. Summer was always a particularly slow time. More than once, when we were in these doldrums and contemplating with dread how we would explain to the troops why we couldn't make payroll, Shubh saved the day by getting on the phone to customers to plead for an advance payment on our work. We usually were only paid upon achievement of pre-specified project milestones. It was highly unusual for any client to pay in advance for work not yet done.

But payroll days were a regular occurrence, milestones were few and far between, and there were times when we simply didn't have enough cash to cover payroll. To his everlasting credit, Shubh was willing, in those lean times, to call in personal favors with his pharma friends and acquaintances. But making these kinds of hat-in-hand calls was always highly stressful, for all of us, but particularly, naturally, for Shubh. Quite rightly, after suffering through such a call, he would march into my office in high dudgeon, announcing that "we've *got* to change the way we do business around here," and slamming his hand down on my desk.

"What do you mean? How do we do business around here?"

He'd roll his eyes and sigh in exasperation. "We are stuck in the mud! If we keep on doing what we're doing, we'll keep on getting what we're getting!"

"What do you mean? What are we doing? What are we getting?"

"All ... the ... *wrong* ... things!" he said, enunciating each word very slowly and deliberately. "We've *got* to give the client what *he* wants, not what *we* want. We have got to change our approach!"

I would respond defensively: "What do you mean? I refuse to produce junk for clients just because they ask for it!"

"That's my point. You should *know* what they really need, even if they don't."

"I'm not a mind reader, Shubh. I don't have a crystal ball! I can't help it if these guys won't tell us what their problems really are, or what they're really trying to accomplish ..."

"Yes, you *can* know that. You *should* know that. And do you know why? Because the purpose of a business is to create and keep its customers! Last time I looked, MetaWorks was supposed to be a *business*, not a lifestyle!"

"Some lifestyle!" I muttered, thinking my eighty hour work weeks didn't feel like the path to ultimate happiness.

Since "what we were getting" never matched our expectations, we tried, again and again, to figure out what our obtuse clients really needed, despite what they *said* they wanted. Maybe then 'what we were getting" would improve. But I wasn't a very good oracle. So, to improve on "what we were getting", we decided to try to change "what we were doing". We decided to try our luck with another so-called health care stakeholder (i.e., not pharma). We decided to be opportunistic, and test the waters with a clinical practice guidelines group. Maybe *this* would be our big breakout chance.

Guidelines developers should have certainly wanted to use our services to build systematic reviews to inform their guidelines, or how else could they expect doctors and clinics to actually believe and follow them? Did they really hope to promulgate guidelines that weren't based on the best available evidence? Of course not (or so we thought).

So Shubh and I flew to the other coast to meet our beta test client. We approached their corporate offices, which were, disconcertingly, located behind locked doors with peepholes. There were no windows and no identifying signs, so matching the suite number with the address on an e-mail they'd sent to Shubh, we knocked tentatively on the closed door. I half expected to hear shouts about disturbing the "Great and Terrible Oz," but instead, the peephole lit up, and a muffled woman's voice called out, "Who is it?"

Shubh called out our names and company.

"Are we expecting you?"

Shubh laughed, "I sure hope so! Ask your boss!"

After a silent pause, she noisily fumbled with a series of locks and opened the door.

"Are we in the right place?" Shubh asked, pointing at the letter he held in his hand.

She nodded, unsmiling.

"Why the peepholes and all the locks?"

"Well, we like the extra security."

She hurried back to her desk, clearly not wanting to discuss it with us.

A bear of a man, who looked and sounded eerily like the late comedian John Candy, lumbered toward us in the reception area. Shubh extended his hand.

"Hi! Are you Mike? We're very impressed with all your security! But why do you need it?"

Mike smiled down on us and shook our hands. "Please come with me," he said, as he ushered us into a dark and windowless meeting room and closed the door behind us. "We had to take precautions. You'll understand. We've had some death threats that we're taking very seriously."

Shubh and I glanced at each other, unable to disguise our genuine surprise. It had never occurred to us that this might be a hazardous job!

"Really? What for?"

"Well, it seems some people don't like our guidelines.

It's because their HMOs use them to deny care—to save money, of course. The HMOs are not *supposed* to use them for that, but they do. We always put disclaimers on our publications that we are offering only 'best case scenarios,' but somehow that often gets lost at implementation, and it seems some of our HMO customers really do deny care. Recently, a patient was kicked out of a hospital too early after surgery and died. The HMO said it was following our suggested post-op length of stay for this procedure, so some relatives of the man who died went on the warpath. The case reached the *New York Times*. Since then, we've been getting death threats over the phone and in the mail."

"Wow! That must be tough for your staff!" Shubh sympathized.

"So what do you think we can do for you?"

"Well, we've been trying to get with the evidence-based medicine movement anyway. This is really just another good reason for us to get serious about it sooner rather than later. So we wanted to talk with you about having MetaWorks provide the evidence we need to back up our guidelines."

Here I jumped in with what I thought was pure and simple common sense.

"But that's backwards. I mean, shouldn't you use the evidence to develop the guidelines in the first place, and not to try to find evidence that supports guidelines after the fact?"

Mike raised his eyebrow. "Really? Is that how you see it?"

Again, Shubh and I glanced at each other in surprise. None of this was going as expected.

Mike continued. "The problem we face is that over 90 percent of medical practice has no published evidence to back it up. It's just accepted practice. So if we only used what's published in the literature to develop guidelines, there wouldn't be any most of the time."

"Good point," I conceded, "but Tom Chalmers would've said we just need to do more randomized trials!"

"Well, until all those trials get done, we need *some* kind of evidence. So for that, we look at best practices in the real world, like at the Mayo Clinic, and then we try to find corroborating evidence in the literature. It's not perfect, but it's the best we can do. But this is very time consuming for us, and we thought if a credible third party did up the evidence for us, the guidelines might be more defensible."

Ah ha! Now it was clear! He wanted us to build him a bulletproof shield of evidence. One we couldn't deliver. Formal studies simply do not exist for the vast majority of patient care decisions. Non-physicians are still surprised to learn this, but it's a reality that doctors learn early on. That is why the practice of medicine is and will remain as much an art as a science. And that art cannot be codified; it must be learned over many years of medical school, residency, and practice. Where evidence leaves off, art picks up. We could assemble bits and pieces of evidence for them, but we couldn't give them the art to fill in the gaps in the shield. The guideline business never panned out for us. So we turned around and tried a different tactic. Namely, we decided to stick with pharma but offer something completely different.

25. "The Customer Is Always Right!" (or *Is* He?)

To stay in the pharmaceutical sector but to offer something quite different, we decided to explore ways to partner with other vendors to better utilize our clinical data hub. High on the list of those other vendors were companies that were modeling clinical trials—or trying to. In architecture, aeronautics, and engineering, simulation and computer-assisted design are integral to most endeavors. Why not in medicine? Why not in clinical research? In the late 1990s, attempts were made to do just that. The equations and the programming required were extensive but doable. The missing ingredient for success was good clinical data to feed the models.

At MetaWorks, we were sitting on a treasure trove of good clinical data, so maybe we could work together with a modeling company. Hence, our trip to California, to visit a well-funded group of brilliant modelers who had succeeded in predicting results of Phase 1 studies, which typically measure absorption, distribution, excretion, and metabolism of drugs at various doses. These measures are more readily quantifiable and predictable, because the mechanistic understanding of how chemicals impact the healthy human organism is often far greater than our clinical understanding of disease. But this did not deter our potential collaborators, or us, from wanting to try to use our clinical data to model efficacy and safety outcomes of Phase 2 and Phase 3 studies.

So off we trekked to the "left coast" once again. We took our new genius friends to lunch at a "Mediterranean" restaurant in Palo Alto that they had recommended. In Southern California, "Mediterranean" apparently means Middle Eastern, for the menu was all falafel and hummus and shawarma. The restaurant was empty; it was still very early for lunch, but not for our East Coast stomachs. Our waitress seemed surprised to see us, but approached tentatively. I suspected she was really the kitchen help, and not a waitress, as she wore a white, heavily food-stained shirt and dirty apron over a black skirt. Broad in the beam and middle-aged, with neglected teeth and a nervous smile, she was definitely not Shubh's typical fencing partner.

"Yes? Are you here to eat?"

"Yes, we *are* here to eat! I'd like the lamb shawarma, but without the pita bread. Can I get that?" he asked matter-of-factly, pointing to the fixed price combo meal on the menu.

Our waitress, looking puzzled, not sure of her English, but clearly trying to please, suggested carefully: "Then maybe you should just have the lamb plate, sir," pointing to another item on the menu.

"No, because then I have to pay for rice and all those vegetables that I don't really want, so why should I pay for them! " Shubh beamed at her, fully expecting her to grant him exactly what he wanted.

But she just smiled back and couldn't seem to find anything to say except a puzzled, "Huh?"

So Shubh explained, speaking very slowly. "Can't you just give me this fixed price meal of lamb shawarma, but leave out the pita bread? "

"But that comes *with* the pita bread. It's automatic.

I can't make a shawarma without the bread. Then it's no longer a shawarma."

"Can you not give me just the lamb and not the bread?"

"I don't think so sir … but I'll check."

She was no longer smiling. This day was not starting out so well for her. As she turned back toward the kitchen, Shubh rolled his eyes and snapped the menu closed. After five minutes, she returned with an older man, distinguished-looking, with a no-funny-business look on his face. He introduced himself as the owner.

The entire conversation was repeated over again, but then Shubh added: "I think I've just given you a new product idea, yes?"

"What do you mean, sir?" the proprietor asked icily.

"You should *pay* me for this great idea, don't you think?"

"No, I do not follow you, sir."

Shubh gave up, and said once more, with obvious exasperation: "Can I just have the lamb shawarma, but without the pita bread?"

The man just shook his head, and said, "We'll see what we can do." He and the woman turned back to the kitchen.

"Well, at least he's showing he can be flexible" Shubh smiled at the rest of us. We had already placed our uncomplicated orders and had received our food.

"Go ahead, eat! Don't wait for me!"

Minutes later, the waitress returned with a big smile, and a plate heaping with lamb shawarma filling and no pita bread. Shubh congratulated her. "See? I *knew* you could do it! Thank you!"

She was clearly pleased and was beaming too. But it was not over.

Shubh took one fork-full of his lamb and started to eye my pita bread, served as a side with my Caesar salad. He said to me, "This dish is really heavy on the onions. I'm starting to think I made a mistake, and I really *do* need to order the pita bread."

"Oh, man!" I said. "Just take mine if you need some!"

He smiled. "Okay. Thanks!"

And he helped himself to my pita bread. When that ran out, he called over the waitress, and said, "You know what? Can I have some pita bread after all?"

She rolled her eyes, sighing "yi-yi-yi."

She stomped into the kitchen, and she returned with the bread and the owner right behind her, shaking his head while smiling at Shubh. "I *told* her you were weird!"

"Weird? Don't you know the customer is *always* right? I just changed my mind, and I really *do* want the bread after all. Thank you so much! Yes, this is really how you should be serving this dish. Lamb shawarma *with* the pita bread. Don't you agree?"

As they headed back for the kitchen, shaking their heads in disbelief, Shubh turned to us and commented: "Don't they know the customer is *always* right?"

By now I had my doubts, and thought of MetaWorks' experience with some of our pharma customers.

"I'm not so sure about that!"

Our modeler friends just laughed, but the exchange

seemed to be emblematic of our attempts to forge a useful working relationship with the modelers. They had the pita bread, and we had the lamb filling, but we couldn't see a way to make it all work together at the same time. So another door to opportunity shut on us.

26. "Be Still, My Heart!"

Our next foray was to find other data sources, beyond what was in the published literature, to supplement and extend our menu of MetaWorks offerings. This time we were intrigued by medical transcription companies that claimed to have a way to "database" all the transcriptions. Traditionally, when doctors see patients, they dictate notes to the patient's medical chart. These dictations are typed up by typing services (transcription companies), corrected by the physicians, and then inserted as part of the patient's permanent medical record. If there was a way to standardize the information in these text notes, to deconstruct it into its component parts, and then to reconstruct those parts into a database, data elements could theoretically be pooled across patients, and analyzed. If this could be done, then this would be an incredibly valuable data source to monitor and measure health care processes and outcomes.

So we flew to Tennessee to "kick the tires" of one such transcription company. After a very long day of mutual show-and-tell at this company, I was bone-weary. Shubh remained chipper, and, of course, he had been slipping into his Southern drawl all day. We entered the ticketing area of the airport, and I immediately scouted out the airline kiosk to get boarding passes for our e-tickets. But Shubh held back. He was eyeing the airline ticket counter agents, and he had spotted someone he was already smiling and nodding at. I looked over to see a friendly-looking, middle-aged woman smiling back and beckoning us to her.

"Shubh, here's the kiosk. Let's just get our boarding passes and go to security."

"No, let's mosey on over heaah to this heaah agent."

"Why? We can do it right here. We're not checking any bags."

"Because I'd *always* rather deal with a real person than a machine! Hi, Pam!" he oozed, spotting her name tag in a nanosecond. "How *aaarrre* you?"

"Why, I'm just fine! And how are you?" Pam beamed.

"I'm just wonderful, now that I've met you!"

"Oh, be still my heart!" she said, as she placed her hand over her heart. While Shubh howled with delight, she added: "Now, what can I do for y'all today?"

"Well, my dear, if you *really* care, you can give us great seats on your flight to Providence, or ... you can invite us home for dinner at your house tonight."

"Well now, I'm not so sure which to do!"

Shubh continued: "Or you could come with us! I suppose hubby might mind, though?"

"Oh, it doesn't matter what he thinks! But the airline really needs me to stay here tonight. I've got to finish my shift!"

"What a shame! I guess we'll just have to go home without you then!"

"Sorry about that! I just know we'd have a lot of fun, but y'all have a wonderful flight now, y'hear?"

"Yes, ma'am, we *shaah* will!"

Variations on this exchange happen whenever we encounter strangers who are willing to play the game. I used to think that this type of behavior would surely offend people. But to my never-ending amazement, it doesn't—at least not when Shubh is the instigator. He somehow gains their unspoken and immediate permission, and the game begins.

I remember one cold and grey Philadelphia morning not long afterwards. It was the last Saturday before Christmas. Everyone was tired of work and ready for the holiday to begin. But instead of Christmas shopping at home with our families, Shubh and I were trying to get into a national hematology conference to meet some clients. We encountered a grim-faced, middle-aged woman sitting like a tank behind the meeting registration desk. She announced that I could pay twelve hundred dollars, and Shubh could pay eight hundred dollars, for entry passes to the meeting.

Shubh smiled brightly at her, noting: "That's incredibly expensive for just one day. The good doctor and I are here just for today. You're not going to make us pay so much for just one day. are you?"

"Yes, I am." She was way too smug.

"Isn't there some way we can qualify for lower rates?"

"No, there's not."

"Aw, c'mon. How about if I go in as a student or a technical assistant? I *can* be that, if I need to be, you know." Shubh smiled broadly.

She hesitated. "Well, I guess so, but she'll still have to pay twelve hundred dollars," she said, pointing at me.

"Okay, let's register me first, as a technical assistant. That's two hundred dollars, right?"

"Um hum," she said, as she completed the paper work and handed him his entry badge.

While pinning it on, he continued: "Okay. Now, let's say the good doctor here is my spouse. Can she attend with me, for a reduced rate?" Again, he was smiling broadly, knowing the answer.

"Why, yes, she can attend as your 'spouse-guest,' for an extra fifty dollars!" The woman was now smiling broadly, seeing in a flash what had just happened. And she added appreciatively: "You are baaaaad news, man!"

"Oh, be still my heart!" Shubh crooned, patting his chest.

She let out a rich, deep belly laugh, as she processed my entry badge.

"Now *that's* creative problem solving!" Shubh slapped the counter for emphasis. "You have a Merry Christmas!"

"I will! And y'all have a nice day now!" She was smiling happily as we walked away.

We never proceeded with the transcription database idea, largely because the database did not exist anywhere except in the heads of the transcription company executives. As we found again and again in our search for good clinical data, there was often much hype, but little reality.

Finally, however, we found what we were looking for—Electronic Medical Record (EMR) data, which hadn't even existed in any useful form when we started MetaWorks. This data source was just gaining traction in the United States in the late 1990s, as a critical mass of physicians adopted these systems to hold their medical chart data. Even when de-identified and anonymized, as it always was for analysis purposes, a patient's medical chart contains a level of clinical detail not previously accessible for research analyses. The best real-world clinical data we could get before EMRs were data on medical payment claims histories from government sources (e.g., Medicare) or private vendors (e.g., UnitedHealthcare). Claims data were better than nothing, particularly for answering questions about payments for care over time, but of little value for clinically important questions of effectiveness or safety of therapeutics in real-world settings. For these sorts of questions, EMR analyses *could* be superb.

Shubh, with sheer bulldog tenacity, brokered a first relationship with an oncology EMR database vendor, which led to several lucrative pharma contracts for MetaWorks. The EMR analysis opened up a wider pharma market for us: one with different clients asking different questions—questions that needed more than published clinical trials to answer. It was a line of business that worked well for MetaWorks. It fit our staff's capabilities and our client's needs, and it yielded a much needed boost in revenues. Finally, we had managed to diversify. Our little fish hadn't learned to fly, but it had arrived in a bigger pond.

27. "We Are All Spiritual Beings Having a Human Experience"

January 2003. We're in a taxi in Manhattan.

Shubh says to the driver: "How are you doing, my good man?" He glances at the driver's ID plate on the back of the seat. "Are you Italian?"

Driver: "No, my first name is Italian—Gennaro—but my mother is Spanish and totally white, and my father is Dominican and totally black. He's darker than me and you put together. I was born in Dominican Republic, but I lived in NYC most of my life."

Shubh: "You don't say? How do you like it?"

Driver: "It's okay. You wouldn't believe all I've learned here."

Shubh: "Like what?"

Driver: "Like where to eat, what to eat, what to do; you know … that kind of stuff."

Shubh: "You should write a book!"

Driver: "Well, I went to college for two years, but I only wrote one research paper. I can't write a book. I need someone like you to give me ideas."

Shubh: "Why don't you go back to school?"

Driver: "Ha! When I win the Lotto! Then I'll buy an apartment on the Upper East Side and go back to school after taking a year off just for fun."

We reach our destination—no more than a few blocks away. Shubh pays him, and ends with this comment: "Well, Gennaro, I hope you find a way to write that book! Thank you, my friend."

The driver smiles and says: "Thank *you!*"

Shubh says to me, as we walk into the restaurant:

"See?　We learned about what really matters to that young man. And he *liked* telling us. After all, we're *all* spiritual beings, having a human experience.　If you just treat people like human beings, they behave like human beings!"

That evening, we dine with our guest, a physician who is very Upper East Side, with a big consulting income and lots of spare time.　She is living our cabbie's dream.　Yet this model of success makes a confession to Shubh after a few glasses of wine. With an embarrassed smile, she declares: "My personal dream is to own a café on the Jersey shore.　Who'da thunk it?"

Shubh beams. "Really? Well, we all have dreams. We're all spiritual beings having a human experience, yes?" He continues: "You know, I've got a dream like that too."

He proceeds to describe his dream of "retirement," in which he will own a whole block of stores on Main Street, USA, probably in one of those lovely little bedroom communities around Boston.　He will own a coffee shop, a dry cleaner, and a gas station.　He will stroll through town each morning, stopping first at his coffee shop, where he will tarry as long as it takes to read the newspaper and sip a tall coffee.　Then he will fold up his paper and move on to his dry cleaner shop.

"How's business, Frank?" he will say.

"Great, Mr. Shubh," Frank will respond.

"Wonderful! Keep up the good work!" will be Shubh's response, as he continues down the street to his gas station, where the same conversation will occur.　It will be a scene straight out of *It's a Wonderful*

Life, before Mr. Potter takes over. Then Shubh will head home and go online to play with his stock portfolio for a few hours. He will probably make more money in this "retirement" than at any other time in his life, and he will be happier than ever!

After dinner, and following the general approval of all retirement dreams, we stop at the coat-check counter, and yet another Shubh moment occurs. He slides his plastic tag across the counter to the coat check girl, saying "I'm 27."

"Is that your age or your check number?" she smiles.

Not missing a beat, Shubh beams. "Will you marry me?"

"Absolutely! But we'll need to have a house in my homeland."

"Nooooo problem! Where's that?"

"Italy, in my mama's village, on the heel of the boot of Italy."

"Like I said, no problem!"

He's now stretching out his arms toward the coat check girl—for a hug, or for his coat, we never find out, because the coat check girl grabs the wrong coat. She hands him the coat belonging to our well-heeled dinner guest. Shubh laughs and points.

"That's hers. She's the rich one!"

The coat check girl clearly admires the sumptuous, full-length shearling coat.

"It was a gift," our guest admits, almost apologetically, as our coat-check girl turns back to Shubh.

"I take it back … I'm going to go home with *her* instead!"

"Oh well, if that's how you feel … it was beautiful while it lasted, my dear!"

And with a tip of his cap, he says, "Have a great night!"

And as we exit, he shakes his head and says, "New Yorkers! Now *they're* spiritual beings!"

The next day, we're heading back to Boston on the Acela Express. This is a great train for firing up a whole lot of Shubh-isms, for it is a place where strangers talk to each other freely. The table seating for four definitely invites conversations. Within two minutes of sitting down across from two young e-traders, Shubh is already past the introductions. The conversation goes like this:

Shubh: "So did you have a good day today?"

Both: "Yes!"

Shubh: "So when you die, what will you tell your Maker you did to improve mankind?"

e-trader #1, not missing a beat: "It's too early to answer that question …I'm only a third of the way done. I don't have time to think about the 'big-purpose' stuff."

e-trader #2: "Well, I helped my clients make some great deals today … all four of them."

Shubh: "Clients or deals?"

e-trader #2: "Deals! Ha! Ha!"

Shubh: "Business is slow?"

e-trader #2: "Yes, business is slow right now."

As the train pulls into a station in coastal Connecticut, e-trader #2 says his good-byes and hurries off the train.

We pull out of the station, and Shubh continues

to press e-trader #1 for details of his life. We learn, in short order: (1) He is adopted from Nebraska, but grew up in Connecticut, (2) he is probably Norwegian and Irish biologically, (3) he is married, no children yet … not ready yet to sacrifice eight hours sleep a night, (4) his wife is a columnist for a small Connecticut newspaper, (5) they each commute daily one hour in different directions to work—he to Manhattan, she to Hartford, (6) she works 4:00 p.m. to midnight, and he works from 9:00 a.m. to 5:00 p.m., so they rarely see each other, and (7) she leaves homemade dinners for him to heat up and eat alone when he gets home each evening.

Shubh: "Give me your card, young man. You seem to be very hardworking and moldable."

e-trader #1: "Ha! My wife is doing all the 'molding' right now, and she's doing a good job."

Shubh: "Yes, I think she is. You are definitely a human *doing*, not just a human *being*."

e-trader#1 gathers his things to exit, as we approach the next station.

e-trader #1: "It was great talking with you. I'll be thinking about my purpose in life, so I'll be ready to answer the Maker's question when we next meet."

Shubh: "You do that, young man. It was a pleasure."

28. Epilogue

In 2006, MetaWorks was bought by a global CRO that wanted a more cerebral identity, an identity that niche consultancies like ours might provide. We had weathered countless storms, as well as doldrums, and suffered our fair share of navigational challenges, mutinous crew, sea monster clients, and low rations. It was a blessed relief to finally bring our little ship to dock. The acquisition allowed those of us who wanted to disembark to finally do so, without jeopardizing our crew members who wished to remain on board. It gave those employees a chance, in a larger, more secure organization, to advance and extend professionally. It was perfect in that regard.

On the other hand, however, the new parent organization swallowed up MetaWorks, and in time, virtually obliterated our original identity and mission. I suppose this was to be expected, as it gradually became clear to me that the traditional CRO business was the top dog in that organization, and we were just a nubbin of a tail attached to that dog. I had dreamed that MetaWorks might be the tail that wagged the dog, but it was not to be. The big revenue makers in the organization seemed to call the shots, and those individuals were clearly not from our little group of nerdy analysts sitting up in Boston.

Still, I'd like to think that, in its time, MetaWorks influenced the healthcare information field in a good way. We were definitely "human-doings." The principles and methods of Evidence-based Medicine continue to evolve in all sectors in health care. And thoughts of Shubh continue to bring smiles to people scattered across companies, across the world. While everyone contributed in his or her own unique way to the successful voyage of the SS MetaWorks, Shubh, through his buoyant sense of fun, kept us afloat.